Fit Buddies to Fit Champs

Journey of Fitness, Friendship & Fun

Aryan Mohan

Qurate
quratebooks.com

Fit Buddies to Fit Champs
Journey of Fitness, Friendship & Fun.
Aryan Mohan

Published in 2024

© Published by

Qurate Books Pvt. Ltd.
Goa 403523, India
www.quratebooks.com
Tel: 1800-210-6527, Email: info@quratebooks.com

ISBN: 978-93-58984-73-6

To all the fitness enthusiasts who dare to dream and strive for more, who inspire each other every day to push boundaries to grow together—this journey belongs to us!

Acknowledgements

This book is a reflection of the unwavering support, love, and encouragement from the incredible people in my life.

To my grandparents, whose unwavering support and guidance continue to motivate me from beyond. Your legacy of strength and perseverance lives on in every step of this journey.

To my parents —your wisdom, guidance, and unwavering belief in me have shaped the person I am today and to my in-laws - your kindness and encouragement have made me feel like one of your own.

To my incredible wife, Mrinalini, your patience, understanding, and boundless love have been my rock. You've stood by me through thick and thin, celebrated every milestone, and have always been my greatest inspiration.

To my children, Niharika and Maahika, your joy, curiosity, and energy bring light into my world. You've taught me the importance of balance and perseverance, and this book is as much yours as it is mine.

To my guardian sisters, Malar and Arul, your love and laughter have lifted me through tough times. Thank you for always cheering me on and being my constant support.

To my brother in laws, Abhi and Anish - I'm deeply grateful for your constant support and love and to my nieces and nephews, Rani, Rahul, Hridishtitha, and Hrishaan - your friendly conversations and fun times have created wonderful memories that I cherish deeply.

To my friends and gym buddies, thank you for being my sounding board, my safe space, and my endless source of motivation. Your camaraderie and shared sense of determination have been a true source of balance.

A heartfelt thank you to the entire team at Qurate Books. To the Founder CEO, Dr. Pramod Khera, your leadership and vision have profoundly shaped this book into what it is today. To my Editor, Milind Jakati, your insightful feedback, meticulous attention to detail, and unwavering dedication have truly brought out the best in this work. I also want to express my gratitude to my Designer Lynessa for her tireless efforts on the book cover; your suggestions and design were both refined and contemporary. To Jonely, whose hard work and dedication to formatting this book is deeply appreciated. I couldn't have accomplished this without each of your invaluable contributions.

I am deeply grateful for each of you being a part of this journey.

Fit Buddies are the stepping stones;
Fit Champs are the milestones!

About the Author

Allow me to introduce myself. My journey has been as diverse as it has been enriching. I graduated from Madurai Kamaraj University, where I was honoured to be a university rank holder. This academic achievement was just the beginning of my foray into the world of learning and excellence. My educational journey continued at IIM Ahmedabad, where I delved deep into the intricacies of management and strategy.

For 16 years, I traversed the corporate world, gaining experience in various roles and industries. From BFSI to wildlife photography, consulting to soft-skills training, followed by my stint into the world of Information Technology, my career has been a kaleidoscope of experiences.

But amidst these professional endeavours, my passion for fitness and writing never waned. These twin passions are deeply rooted in my childhood, shaped by extensive travel and the myriad of experiences that come with it.

Preface

The journey to fitness is never walked alone. It's a collective experience marked by shared challenges, mutual support, and the joy of achieving goals together. In this book, I—Aryan—invite you to walk with me on a transformative journey that started with me as a humble 'Fit Buddy' and led to my evolution into a 'Fit Champ'.

In the beginning, I was just one of many at the gym, a face in the crowd, offering nods of recognition to fellow fitness enthusiasts. Like many, I believed that fitness was all about the individual challenge: how much weight I could lift, how far I could run, or how fast I could achieve my goals. But what I soon realised was that fitness is far more meaningful when it becomes a shared experience. The Fitness Centre wasn't just a place for personal improvement, it was a space for connection, for shared high-fives after a tough workout, for motivation passed between breaths of exhaustion, and for collective victories celebrated together.

This realisation reshaped my approach to fitness entirely. I began as a Fit Buddy, someone simply present, working through the emotions. But I soon found myself becoming a part of something bigger. Fitness wasn't just my individual journey anymore—it was 'ours'. The encouragement I received from others pushed me harder, and in turn, I found myself supporting those around me. That's when my role began to shift. I was no longer just a participant; I was becoming a mentor, a motivator, and a champion for others.

The path to becoming a Fit Champ wasn't marked by reaching new personal records or standing at the top of a podium. It was about stepping into a role where I could help others find their own strength and potential. Being a Fit Champ meant leading by example, but also cheering others on when they needed it most, sharing in their setbacks and celebrating their progress. It was about building relationships within the fitness community, knowing that each small victory was a win for us all.

This book is not just the story of my fitness journey—it's a reflection of the many individuals who have walked this path with me. It's a testament to the power of teamwork, persistence, and the belief that the journey is always better when experienced together. Through these pages, I hope to offer not only my story but also inspiration to help you achieve your own goals, and perhaps more importantly, to inspire and support those around you on their own fitness journeys.

The vision for this book is simple yet profound: *To inspire lifelong fitness through camaraderie.*

Welcome to the transformation—from Fit Buddy to Fit Champ.

Let's continue to rise, together.

Contents

Introduction **15**

Phase I

BEING A FIT BUDDY **21**

- Tuesday Morning Motivation: A Fresh Start 23
- The Unseen Coach: A Gym Morning's Silent Test 31
- Unlocking the Mystery - Fitness Trainers' Hidden Playbook 39
- Gravity's Challenge: The Balance Breakthrough 45
- Flex It Like a Yogi: Unveiling the Power of Stretching 51
- Sneaker Trap: How One Wrong Choice Left Me Limping 57

Phase II

BEING A FIT CHAMP **63**

- Building Bonds and Breaking Sweat: Embracing Camaraderie at our Fitness Centre 65

- The Shivagange Trek - Part 1: From Dawn to Summit in Hilarious Harmony! 72
- The Shivagange Trek – Part 2: Monkey Business, Treacherous Trails, and Whimsical Wishes 84
- The Shivagange Trek – Part 3: Krishna's Concoction and the Journey Back....................95
- Bruised, Bold, and Blissful: The Fab4's Daredevil Dash Odyssey....................105
- Tee-Rific Triumph: The 5:30 AM Squad's Epic Tee-Shirt Adventure 123
- Embracing Responsibility with a Dash of Fun....................138

Epilogue: The Fitness Journey Continues… 142

Introduction

Welcome to a transformative journey, where fitness meets storytelling, and camaraderie becomes the cornerstone of personal growth. This book is not just about exercise routines and dietary advice; it's a celebration of the human spirit, a tribute to the power of community, and a testament to the joy that comes from leading a healthy and active life.

Fitness is not just about the physical aspect; it's about building a community, fostering relationships, and finding joy in the process. This book is designed to offer you motivation, relatable experiences, and comprehensive fitness knowledge. It encourages the building of supportive fitness communities and fosters resilience to overcome challenges in your fitness pursuits and beyond.

Throughout this book, you will encounter stories that will make you laugh, think, and perhaps even shed a tear. From the early morning motivation sessions to the empowering lessons learned from trainer-free workouts, each chapter is designed to resonate with your own fitness journey.

You will meet individuals who have overcome personal obstacles, embraced new challenges, and found joy in the most unexpected places. Their stories are a testament to the human spirit and a reminder that fitness is not just about the destination but the journey itself.

One of the key themes of this book is the importance of community. Fitness is not a solitary endeavour; it's about building bonds, supporting each other, and finding strength in numbers. Whether it's through the shared experience of a challenging workout, the camaraderie of a fitness group, or the encouragement of a workout buddy, the support of a community can make all the difference.

As you read through the chapters, you will find practical advice on how to build and maintain a supportive fitness community. From organising group workouts to participating in fitness challenges, there are countless ways to foster a sense of belonging and support.

Fitness journeys are seldom smooth sailing. There will be obstacles, setbacks, and moments of doubt. But it is through these challenges that we grow stronger, both physically and mentally. This book is filled with stories of resilience, of individuals who have faced adversity head-on and emerged victorious.

The lessons learned from these experiences are invaluable. They teach us the importance of perseverance, the power of a positive mindset, and the strength that comes from within. As you navigate your own fitness journey, these stories will serve as a source of inspiration and a reminder that you are not alone.

Above all, this book is a celebration of the joy that comes from leading a healthy and active life. Fitness is not just about the physical benefits; it's about finding happiness in the process, enjoying the journey, and embracing the fun along the way. From the exhilarating feeling of a good workout to the laughter shared with workout buddies, the joy of fitness is a powerful motivator.

As you delve into the chapters, you will discover the myriad of ways in which fitness can bring joy to your life. Whether it's through a challenging yoga session, a thrilling trek, or a fun fitness event, the possibilities are endless.

As we embark on this fitness adventure together, I invite you to open your mind and heart to the stories, lessons, and experiences shared in this book. Let them inspire you, motivate you, and guide you on your own fitness journey. Remember, fitness is not just about reaching a goal; it's about enjoying the journey, building bonds, and finding joy in the process.

Whether you are a fitness enthusiast looking for new motivation, a beginner seeking guidance, or someone interested in improving your overall health and well-being, this book has something for you.

So, let's lace up our shoes, embrace the challenge, and embark on this journey together.

Welcome to a world of fitness, camaraderie, and endless possibilities.

Let the adventure begin!

Phase I

BEING A FIT BUDDY

My journey into fitness began with nervous anticipation, much like anyone stepping into a gym for the first time. I wasn't an expert, didn't know the perfect techniques or the proper form for exercises. But what I did have was a willingness to learn, a deep curiosity, and a desire to be part of something larger than myself.

A 'Fit Buddy' is not defined by expertise but by their eagerness to explore the world of fitness as part of a community. It's someone who, despite being new to the gym, embraces the learning process and the opportunity to grow alongside others.

At first, I was just another face in the crowd, standing among seasoned lifters and those who seemed to have mastered the gym environment. The rows of machines, the energetic atmosphere, and the apparent ease with which others navigated their workouts were all a bit overwhelming. I didn't know how to use many of the machines or perform the exercises properly, but I was determined. I approached each workout with humility, eager to observe and learn. I wasn't afraid to make mistakes or ask for advice, knowing that growth came through the process of trial and error.

What made my journey as a Fit Buddy special was my natural inclination to connect with others. I wasn't just there to achieve my own fitness goals—I was there to be part of something bigger. I observed people around me, struck up conversations, and soon those casual nods evolved into shared encouragement and camaraderie. I realised that fitness wasn't just about personal progress, but also about the bonds you form with those on the same path.

As a Fit Buddy, I made it a point to be an active participant in the gym's community spirit. Even though I wasn't an expert, my enthusiasm became contagious. My willingness to try new things, laugh at my own stumbles, and keep pushing forward, made me approachable to others.

In the following chapters, I'll walk you through my early days (Phase I) of being a Fit Buddy where I was full of curiosity and connection. These stories will show you how fitness is as much about the people we surround ourselves with, as it is about personal goals.

Tuesday Morning Motivation: A Fresh Start

It was Feb 7, 2023 and there's something uniquely magical about Tuesday mornings. Maybe it's the way the early light filters through the curtains, or the faint promise of a fresh start, but there's an almost palpable energy in the air. It's on these quiet mornings that I can feel the potential for transformation; where the routine of waking up early and pushing myself can set the tone for the rest of the week. Today, it felt as if the universe was holding its breath, waiting for me to make the first move.

I know that getting out of bed on a chilly Tuesday morning isn't always as invigorating as it sounds. The comfort of my bed can be a fierce adversary, a warm cocoon that wraps around me and whispers sweet nothings of "just five more minutes." I could feel my body rebelling, every fiber of it clinging to the soft, inviting warmth of my bed. My alarm clock seemed to have a vendetta against me, blaring its relentless tune, urging me to rise and shine when all I wanted was to hide under the covers.

This battle wasn't just with my bed; it was a conflict of willpower. Each morning, I was faced with a choice: give in to the seduction of sleep or muster the resolve to get up and start my day. It wasn't about dumbbells or running shoes just yet—it was about wrestling with the inertia of comfort. My blankets seemed to have a life of their own, wrapping me tighter, convincing me that staying in bed would be a perfectly fine decision. But then, in a moment of quiet determination, I swung my legs over the edge of the bed. The cold floor greeted me, a sharp contrast to the cozy warmth I'd just left behind.

There's a subtle victory in those early morning struggles, a triumph of motivation that isn't always visible but is deeply felt. Today, that victory was embodied by me, and I was determined to make it to my fitness center in Bangalore. My morning began with a reluctant rise, a fight against the comfort of his bed, and this struggle was just the beginning.

My day had started with the usual chaos: mismatched socks, a pair of shorts that seemed to have shrunk in the wash, and the nagging thought that maybe a few more minutes of sleep wouldn't hurt. But as I finally stepped out into the world, I was met with an unexpected twist. The skies above had decided to engage in a water-themed extravaganza, turning Bangalore into a rainy spectacle. It was as if someone had opened the floodgates, and rain poured down with the kind of enthusiasm usually reserved for overzealous water balloon fights.

Navigating through the downpour, I arrived at the fitness center, only to be greeted by an unusual sight. The usual buzz of morning activity was absent. The streetlights were flickering weakly, casting eerie shadows that made the scene look like that from a low-budget horror film. The fitness center, usually alive with the hum of treadmills and the clinking of weights, was eerily quiet. It resembled more of an abandoned warehouse than the vibrant hub it usually was.

A quick look around, and it wasn't hard to figure out what had happened. The entire neighbourhood was cloaked in darkness, thanks to a transformer explosion that had taken out the power grid. The usual bright and bustling area had turned into what felt like a blackout bingo, with every street corner contributing to the overarching theme of pitch-black nothingness. The darkness was so complete, so enveloping, that it seemed almost like a scene from a sci-fi movie—a black hole had swallowed the neighbourhood, leaving us stranded in its inky depths.

Yet, in the face of this unexpected obstacle, the morning's usual workout crew began to arrive. They were a determined bunch, as tenacious as caffeinated squirrels, and a power outage wasn't going to stop them from getting their exercise in. Each member arrived clutching their yoga mats, dumbbells, and the kind of resolve you'd expect from people gearing up for a zombie apocalypse, not just a routine morning workout. The group's resilience was infectious; even in the dim light and chilly rain, we found ourselves smiling, laughing, and sharing in the absurdity of the situation.

For about fifteen minutes, we stood outside the gym, waiting for a solution to present itself. The usual cacophony of gym machines was replaced by the rhythmic plink-plunk of raindrops and the occasional rumble of thunder—a soundtrack that seemed almost too perfect for the morning's turn of events. The rain wasn't just falling; it was performing, adding a melodramatic flair to our already surreal circumstances.

But standing in the rain wasn't exactly the workout anyone had in mind. So, we did what any group of motivated individuals would do—we brainstormed. Well, *brainstormed* might be too formal a term. It was more like a lively debate mixed with spontaneous bursts of creativity and humour. Ideas were tossed around with the kind of energy that only comes from facing unexpected adversity together.

Someone suggested we just embrace the rain and hold our session outside.

"Aquatic Burpees, anyone?" another voice chimed in, the suggestion drawing a round of chuckles.

The conversation shifted, each idea more creative and unconventional than the last. A rooftop workout? A session in the nearby park? The energy was contagious, as if the blackout had unlocked some hidden reservoir of creativity within us all. What started as a setback was quickly morphing into an opportunity for something new and exciting—a shared experience that was about more than just fitness; it was about community and the shared spirit of adventure.

Amid all this, our center manager embarked on his own quest. Determined not to let the morning go to waste, he set out on what could only be described as a heroic mission: finding fuel for the backup generator. The image of him braving the rain, dodging puddles, and navigating the morning chaos in search of fuel was almost cinematic—a modern-day knight on a quest not for a holy grail but for the elusive fuel that would save our workout. His journey added a layer of comedy to our morning, a subplot that was as entertaining as the workout session we were about to create.

As we waited, the fitness centre sent out an apology message to its members, offering a two-day membership extension as a kind of consolation prize for the inconvenience. The message was met with mixed reactions. Some members took the extension and headed home, content with the unexpected break. But others, driven by the same determination that had gotten them out of bed in the first place, refused to let the morning end in defeat.

One of the more outspoken members, with the conviction of someone who had just given a motivational speech, declared that leaving now would be tantamount to surrender. The sentiment resonated with many of us—after all, waking up early and braving the rain for a workout meant something. It wasn't just about the exercise; it was about commitment, about not giving up when things didn't go according to plan.

Another member, ever practical, suggested we take the session to her terrace. It wasn't ideal, she admitted, but it was dry, spacious, and better than waiting around in the rain. The idea had a certain appeal, especially since the prospect of a rooftop workout carried its own charm.

I listened, taking in the various suggestions with the focus of someone piecing together a puzzle. Each idea seemed to add a new piece to the unfolding situation, and as I mentally turned each one over, I couldn't help but feel a sense of responsibility to contribute. After all, we were a team, a community, and in moments like these, everyone's input mattered.

The conversation flowed around me, a mix of hopeful suggestions and light-hearted banter, but I was still searching for something that would click, something that would make sense of the chaotic situation we found ourselves in. Finally, as if an internal gear had shifted, two potential scenarios began to form in my mind, each one taking shape with the clarity that comes from listening to the collective brainstorming of a motivated group.

I turned to Avijit, our ever-energetic trainer, whose optimism had become the glue holding our group together through the morning's uncertainty. With a deep breath, I pitched the two ideas that had been swirling in my mind.

The first was a *Terrace Workout*. One of our members had already suggested using their terrace as a backup location. The idea wasn't without its challenges—dodging potted plants, avoiding the occasional dive-bombing pigeon—but it offered a practical solution to our predicament. We could move the workout to the terrace and make the best of the situation, embracing the novelty of an outdoor session in a space that was at least dry and relatively spacious.

The second option was more conventional but equally dependent on a bit of luck—*Gym Revival*. If our center manager, who had heroically ventured out into the rain to procure fuel for the generator, managed to return successful, we could resume our workout in the familiar comfort of the gym. The appeal of functioning equipment and a well-lit space was undeniable, especially given the less-than-ideal weather conditions. It was the safer, more predictable option, but it hinged entirely on whether the fuel could be secured in time.

The third, unconventional option we considered was 'Aquatic Workout' i.e working out in the rain, a suggestion from a member early on, and I could see the excitement building among others, as soon as it was mentioned. Since it wasn't raining too heavily, the group was eager for a change in plans. What amused me next was seeing members crossing their fingers, silently hoping the manager wouldn't return with the fuel for the generator, which would have meant sticking to the original indoor workout. The anticipation for an outdoor session in the rain was clearly winning everyone over.

Avijit, true to his nature, was open to all the ideas. His adaptability had always been one of his strongest traits, and in this moment, it was clear that he was ready to roll with whatever scenario played out. There was something reassuring in his calm acceptance of the situation, a quiet confidence that suggested we'd make the best of things no matter what.

Minutes ticked by, filled with anticipation. Along with the other members, I was waiting anxiously for the outcome of the center manager's fuel run, eyes fixed on the street, hoping for any sign of his return. It was an unusual kind of suspense, turning our otherwise routine morning into an unexpected adventure. The uncertainty kept us on edge but also brought us closer together as a group.

Suddenly, Prateek shouted, "Hey, the manager's coming with the fuel can!"

But instead of excitement, the reaction was more like a collective, "Ohhh man!"

I watched it all unfold, feeling mixed emotions. Part of me was relieved that we'd be able to work out indoors, but another part of me secretly wished for a rain workout—it would be a unique, thrilling experience.

As the manager parked his bike, I noticed he wasn't struggling to carry the fuel can, and I thought, "Wow, he's strong!"

Prateek, who had suggested the rain workout earlier, jokingly said, "Maybe he's carrying an empty can! If we'd followed my idea, we wouldn't have wasted 20 minutes!"

I couldn't help but admire his confidence—he seemed sure that the can was empty and that Avijit would lead us in the rain workout anyway. When the manager approached, I smiled and thanked him for going out in the rain to get the fuel.

He surprised me by saying, "Why are you thanking me? I didn't get any fuel."

I was caught off guard, but Prateek jumped in, "Alright, time for the aquatic workout—let's not waste any more time!"

Avijit, our trainer, nodded in agreement, already on board with the idea. He asked everyone to clear space by moving their motorbikes, and suddenly, the earlier uncertainty transformed into excitement for the rain workout! The energy shifted as we regrouped, ready for what was now dubbed the "Aquatic Workout." This was more than just exercise—it felt like a collective victory. The 40-minute session that followed was unlike anything we'd done before, reminiscent of a Navy SEAL drill, with bodyweight movements and calisthenics in the rain. There was an intensity in the air, a shared determination that made me push harder than usual. Every drop of sweat being washed away by falling raindrops from above, felt more significant, every rep more purposeful.

As we powered through the final moments, I felt a deep sense of pride—not just in myself, but in everyone around me. This wasn't just a workout; it was a shared experience that had turned a potential disaster into something extraordinary. We had come together as a team, each person contributing in their own way, creating a moment that would stick with us for a long time.

When the session finally ended, there was a tangible feeling of accomplishment. I thanked Avijit for his flexibility and positive attitude—his calm leadership in the face of uncertainty kept us all motivated. It was clear that he was more than just a trainer; he was a source of inspiration, someone who could turn even the most unpredictable mornings into something meaningful. I also thanked Prateek for his out-of-the-box thinking and persistence in suggesting the rain workout. It was an idea that ultimately made everyone's day!

The rain continued to fall, but there was no rush or frustration—just a collective sense of satisfaction and acceptance of the unexpected twist the morning had brought.

As we went our separate ways, I pondered the allure of the bed that morning, the soft warmth that had invited me to return and escape the unforeseen challenge. The temptation had been strong, to turn back and let the day be defined by an unexpected rain and a blackout. But I had chosen otherwise.

The resistance hadn't been just from the rain or the damp ground, but it had been from within. It was about confronting the unexpected and continuing regardless. It wasn't just a physical challenge but a mental one, a test of attitude and perspective.

This morning hadn't been merely about exercise; it had been about something deeper, something that had transcended the boundaries of a typical workout session. Today I had not only pushed through physical discomfort; I had embodied a lesson in *resilience*. It was not the kind that comes from the straightforward act of lifting weights or running laps, but a resilience born from the act of showing up despite the odds.

It was in the act of showing up despite the rain, of pushing through discomfort, of adapting to the unexpected.

It was a lesson learned not from words but from the silent act of perseverance.

I now approach problems with a newfound focus on solutions rather than obstacles. Setbacks are no longer discouraging but rather moments to refine my approach, fortify my resolve, build strength and character.

Throughout the day, as I go about my usual tasks, I am constantly reminded of this lesson. Every little thing that crossed my path seems to reinforce the importance of sticking to my routine, especially the need to hit the hay early so I'm ready for the workout awaiting me the next morning.

The lesson of RESILIENCE has become more than just a phrase I repeat—it has become a core part of who I am. It's a truth that doesn't need to be spoken aloud; it's something I feel deeply!

The Unseen Coach: A Gym Morning's Silent Test

The next morning, February 8, 2023, as I walked into the gym for my usual group session, there was the typical pre-workout vibe in the air—a mix of sleepy optimism and mild dread, the kind only the early risers know. I could hear the faint chatter about the latest protein powders or weekend plans as people trickled in, clutching their water bottles like lifelines. For a moment, it felt like just another day, another chance to push our limits and get our sweat on.

But today, the gym had a little surprise up its sleeve. And no, not the good kind, like stumbling upon an extra protein bar in the pocket of your gym bag. No, this was more like stepping into a puddle I didn't see coming—a little jolt to start the day off. Our beloved trainer, Avijit—the guy who could coax an extra set of burpees out of us with nothing more than a stern look—was not to be seen. Rumour spread fast, as it always does in a room full of people itching for an excuse to avoid burpees. Someone mentioned something about a last-minute emergency, and just like that, the atmosphere shifted from "ready to crush it" to "what on Earth do we do now?"

I, along with other members, were standing at the workout arena, looking around at each other, waiting for some sort of direction. It's funny how a room full of motivated, capable adults can suddenly feel completely lost without a designated leader. There was a collective moment of, "Uh, what now?" hanging in the air. It would've been so easy to call it a day, throw in the towel, and head back home to the comfort of our beds. Without Avijit there to keep us in line, who was going to stop this from turning into a chat session, or worse, a nap on the yoga mats?

But this is where resilience kicks in, that sneaky little life lesson that tends to pop up when you least expect it. I can read all the motivational quotes in the world about perseverance and grit, but when I am actually standing in the moment, resilience feels like something much simpler, and much harder to describe. It's not a heroic battle cry; it's more of a quiet, internal decision to just keep going, even when things don't go according to plan.

And that's exactly where I was —standing with others in a room without a leader, faced with a choice. Should I bail? Or should I roll with it and figure out a way to make this work?

The glances I exchanged with others said it all. A few of us including me had that "Well, this is awkward" look, while others seemed like they were already considering making a break for the exit. But something funny happens when a group of people is forced out of their routine: they adapt. The silence was broken by the soft clink of a dumbbell hitting the floor, and before I knew it, there was this unspoken agreement that washed over the members. We didn't need a trainer. We could handle this. We'd been coming to these classes long enough to know the routine. Maybe this was our moment to step up, to prove to ourselves that we didn't need someone guiding us to make it through a workout.

Luckily, we had a secret weapon: the Fitness Centre app. This little gem is like having a personal trainer, except it's in my pocket, and it wouldn't make me feel guilty when I decide to skip leg day. No judgment, just a simple, effective guide through every squat, lunge, and plank. The app is more of a no-nonsense coach—it won't hype me up or tell me to "dig deep", but it'll make sure I know what I am doing without turning it into a big production. Need a demo of how to do a burpee without looking like I am having a minor breakdown? The app's got a video for that. Want to make sure my jumping jacks don't devolve into a chaotic arm-flailing dance? It's on it.

The app, isn't just a handy tool—it's a full-blown lifesaver. Instead of guiding us with "Turn left in 500 meters," it's more like, "Here's how to avoid turning that lunge into a full-blown disaster." It's essential, especially for those of us who aren't exactly known for our coordination. And while the app is a fantastic ally, it's not flying solo in this fitness adventure.

Enter our second hero: *the Workout Board*. Picture it as the sacred scroll of fitness wisdom, not just any old whiteboard, but a gospel of sweat etched in dry-erase marker. Each day, the board greets me with the day's exercises, sets, and repetitions, ensuring that I don't wander aimlessly around the gym like a lost soul. It's my workout map, guiding me through the labyrinth of dumbbells and resistance bands. Without it, I'd be like an explorer without a compass, probably found in the corner, staring blankly at the equipment, contemplating if today's the day to finally tackle that weird-looking machine I've been avoiding for months.

But here's the kicker: as amazing as the app and the board are, they come with a tiny caveat. They can't prevent me from making a complete fool of myself in real time. Sure, the app shows me how to do the perfect squat, but it's not going to swoop in and correct my form when my knees start wobbling like a new-born giraffe. And the board? It's not going to throw up a red flag when I mistakenly interpret 'burpees' as "lie flat on the mat and pretend to stretch."

That's not to say I'm not grateful for these tools. Quite the opposite! The app and the board are my dynamic duo, the Batman and Robin of my fitness aids. They keep me on track, ensuring I don't accidentally skip out on the tough stuff (like leg day—ugh) and remind me that, yes, I did sign up for this, and no, lounging in the sauna for 45 minutes doesn't count as a workout. They're the GPS of the gym, guiding me through the wilderness of workouts and making sure I stay on course without too many detours into the "Well, that's close enough" zone.

However, as much as I appreciate these tools, nothing beats having a trainer present to catch all the little mistakes. Without their eagle-eyed supervision, there's always the risk of thinking I'm nailing a move when, in reality, I'm inventing a brand-new exercise that's more interpretive dance than effective workout. Like that one time I thought I'd mastered the deadlift, only to discover I was actually performing some half-bent-over comedy routine. I guess that's why they call it a 'deadlift'—because it nearly killed my dignity.

The thing about fitness is that there's always room for improvement, whether I'm doing squats, lunges, or planks. Sure, the app and the board are fantastic for providing direction, but nothing beats the in-the-moment correction from a trainer. They're the ones who catch me when my form starts to go haywire, remind me to engage my core when all I want to do is collapse into a puddle of sweat, and stop me from turning my workout into a series of unintentional slapstick gags. Standing there, contemplating the gym floor with a growing sense of dread, I had resigned myself to a potential workout disaster.

Then, in a twist, worthy of a superhero origin story, Aashna and Prateek entered the scene. You might know them as regular gym-goers, just like me. They were usually focused on their routines, blending into the gym's backdrop like all the other dedicated fitness enthusiasts. But today, they were about to become the unsung heroes of my workout saga. There were no capes fluttering in the wind or dramatic orchestral scores swelling in the background. It was just Aashna and Prateek, stepping up without any advance notice, and with no fanfare or grand speeches. They simply saw that we were in a bit of a bind and decided to take charge.

I gathered around the workout board along with other members, each of us peering at our phones with the kind of intensity you'd expect from someone trying to solve a Rubik's Cube. The app I usually relied on for guidance was now my lifeline, and I clung to it like it was the last piece of a puzzle. Aashna and

Prateek, though, made this chaotic situation remarkably smooth. They didn't need a script or a rehearsed plan. It was as if they had been waiting for this exact moment, their calm and collected demeanour suggesting they had an innate talent for leading in a pinch.

Aashna was the first to take charge, her easy-going confidence shining through. She demonstrated each exercise with a natural grace that made me wonder if she had missed her calling as a professional trainer. She broke down each move, offering tips that were practical and oddly reassuring. "Engage your core," she'd say, her voice calm and steady. Then came the classic, "Pretend you're not dying inside." It was as if she had a magical ability to turn our nervousness into focus.

Prateek didn't lag behind in enthusiasm. If Aashna was the calm sea, Prateek was the refreshing breeze. His energy was contagious, and his encouragement made even the toughest exercises seem manageable. They were like the personal cheerleaders I never knew I needed, only without the pompoms and awkward high-fives. Their dynamic was almost magical—seamless and effortless, like they were born to do this.

The way they took over was nothing short of inspiring. What could have descended into a chaotic mess of sweaty confusion turned into a workout that felt almost choreographed. It wasn't just a jumble of exercises; it became a rhythm, a flow, a perfectly synchronised routine. It was like a flash mob, but instead of dancing to catchy tunes, I was moving through burpees and squats with a sense of purpose and unity.

By the end of the session, I was buzzing—not just from the endorphins but from the realisation that we had turned a potentially disastrous workout into one of the most satisfying sessions I could remember. The fact that it was far from perfect didn't bother me. What mattered was how Aashna and Prateek had stepped up and showed me that sometimes, the best outcomes come from the most unexpected places.

This experience was more than just a lesson in how to get through a workout without a trainer. It was a masterclass in taking initiative and leadership. Aashna and Prateek didn't have all the answers, and they weren't trained professionals, but they had something even more valuable: the willingness to step up and make the best of a tough situation. It was a powerful reminder that greatness often emerges when you least expect it.

As I packed my gym bag and slung it over my shoulder, ready to head out, a surprising realisation dawned on me. It wasn't just the satisfying ache in my muscles or the endorphin-fuelled glow of a killer workout; it was something deeper, something that hit me as I took that final look around the gym. Today, I learned an unexpected lesson about TRUST.

Now, I'm not talking about the kind of trust where you hope your workout buddy won't drop a barbell on your chest. No, today's lesson was about a deeper, more fundamental kind of trust—the kind that plays a huge role not just in the gym, but in life. It's the trust that lets you lean on others, even when you're not sure how things will turn out.

If I recall correctly, today's workout was supposed to be a well-oiled machine, with our trainer guiding the members through every move, ensuring that we stayed on track and didn't end up face down on the floor after an ill-fated burpee. But as it turned out, our trainer had taken an unscheduled leave, leaving us with no official leader, no badges, no whistles—just Aashna and Prateek, two gym-goers who had suddenly found themselves in charge.

At first, I'll admit, I was a little skeptical. I had shown up expecting the usual routine, led by someone who knew exactly what they were doing. Instead, I was faced with a big question mark. But then, Aashna and Prateek stepped up. There wasn't a dramatic fanfare or a grand announcement; they just took charge with a quiet confidence that, honestly, was pretty reassuring.

I could see it in everyone's eyes: a mix of hesitation and hope. I am used to relying on the trainer for guidance, for motivation, for making sure I don't accidentally turn a squat into a dance move. Now, without that familiar structure, I had to rely on Aashna and Prateek. It wasn't something that happened instantly. Trust began to build slowly, like the gym lights flickering on after a power outage. I started to realise that even though the duo weren't certified trainers, they were here to help us through this. And sometimes, that's all it takes.

There was something almost magical about the way they took over. They weren't trying to revolutionise our workout or introduce some avant-garde fitness philosophy. Their goal was simple: to make sure we didn't flounder in the chaos. Trusting them wasn't about relinquishing control; it was about recognising that I didn't have to do everything by myself. It was about leaning into the collective energy of the group and understanding that all the members had something to contribute.

As the workout progressed, the trust I placed in Aashna and Prateek wasn't just about making sure the session didn't fall apart. It was about realising that when I trust others, I open myself up to new possibilities. I had no idea how things would turn out, but as I followed their lead, something remarkable happened. The workout, which could have been a complete mess, started to flow. I moved through each exercise with a sense of purpose, and every so often, Aashna or Prateek would offer a tip or encouragement that kept me on track.

We were all in this together, and that sense of teamwork was palpable. It wasn't just about Aashna and Prateek leading us; it was about us supporting each other, pushing through, and making sure that no one was left behind. We formed an unspoken pact, a collective promise that we'd make it through the session, no matter what.

This wasn't just a lesson in teamwork; it was a reminder that trust isn't reserved for the big moments, like letting someone spot you during a heavy lift. It's also about the small things—trusting that Aashna and Prateek would guide me through a workout that could have easily spiralled into chaos. It's about believing that even though today's class wasn't what I expected, it would still be worth my time and effort.

And honestly, it was. By the time we finished, I wasn't just proud of the workout I'd done. I was amazed at how well everything had come together once I let go of our initial doubts. I didn't need perfection; I just needed to trust them and believe that together, we could make it work. And we did.

As I walked from the exit, still buzzing from the workout, I realised that today's session had been more than just a spontaneous sweat session. It was a masterclass in focus, trust, confidence, and collaboration, sprinkled with a dash of "Let's wing it and see what happens!"

Since that day, my perspective has changed w.r.t the way I approach professional and personal life. TRUST has allowed me to handle situations at office and at home with more ease, knowing that I don't have to carry the weight of everything alone. By leaning on each other's strengths, we've achieved outcomes far beyond what I could have accomplished on my own!

This newfound reliance on others has been a game-changer, making my journey in both areas more rewarding and collaborative. Now, I see how shared efforts, built on trust, gives a nurturing creative space and freedom to others, thus leading to better results!

Unlocking the Mystery - Fitness Trainers' Hidden Playbook

On Feb 9, 2023, the blaring of my alarm at 4:15 a.m. had become a familiar and even comforting sound, the signal that it was time to start another day. Yet, today, as the loud beeping echoed in my room, I felt a strange hesitation, an unfamiliar weight keeping me anchored to my bed. Usually, I would spring up without a second thought, eager to dive into my morning routine and head to the gym, but not today. Instead, I found myself lying there, staring blankly at the ceiling, torn between the familiar warmth of my blanket and the lingering chaos of yesterday's gym session.

Yesterday had thrown me off balance. Our trainer hadn't shown up—a rarity that disrupted the structure I relied on to guide me through the workout. The sudden absence of that familiar leadership left me uncertain and confused. But in the midst of that disarray, something unexpected had happened. Aashna and Prateek, two of my fellow gym members, had stepped up and taken charge. They had guided us through the session with an ease and confidence I had never seen before. And remarkably, it had worked! Not only did we get through the workout, but we also had fun. There was an energy in the room, a sense of camaraderie that made the session more enjoyable than usual.

Still, the unpredictability of it all left me unsettled. What if the trainer didn't show up again today? Could I handle another day of improvisation? Or worse, what if no one stepped up to lead this time? As these questions swirled through my mind, I found myself frozen in place, unable to move. Part of me admired Aashna and Prateek for their leadership, but another part of me was anxious. The idea of taking the lead myself seemed overwhelming. Could I really guide an entire class through a workout? What if I failed?

I glanced at the clock. It was already 4:45 a.m. If I didn't get up soon, I'd miss the class. The idea of skipping it gnawed at me, but so did the thought of facing the unpredictability of the situation. What if today was as chaotic as yesterday? What if, I had to take the lead and I wasn't ready?

With a sigh, I finally threw off the blanket and forced myself to get up. As I rushed through my morning routine, brushing my teeth and pulling on my workout clothes, I couldn't shake the feeling of uncertainty. I wasn't sure what I was walking into today, but something inside me refused to let me skip the class. The idea of missing out, of not showing up, felt worse than whatever unpredictability awaited me at the gym.

As I made my way to the gym, the questions kept spinning in my mind. Would this roller-coaster ride of unpredictability become the new normal? Or would things return to the steady routine I had grown so accustomed to? And even more pressing—could I find the strength to step up if needed?

When I finally walked through the gym doors, I felt a wave of relief. Our trainer was there, standing confidently at the front of the room, just like always. I hadn't realized how much I had come to rely on that steady presence. There was something deeply comforting about having a leader who knew exactly what to do, who could guide us through even the most challenging workouts with ease and assurance. It wasn't just about the exercises themselves; it was about the sense of stability that came from knowing someone was in control, someone who showed up day after day, no matter what.

Yet, yesterday had been a revelation. It wasn't just the trainer who made the gym function; it was the entire community. Aashna and Prateek had proven that leadership could come from anyone. Even in the absence of the official leader, someone could step up and guide us. Still, as I began to stretch and warm up, I found myself reflecting on what made the trainers different. It wasn't just their expertise or their ability to lead a class—it was their consistency. They showed up every day without fail, and that reliability inspired me. It was their discipline, their unwavering commitment, that kept me and the others coming back.

As I moved through the warm-up, my mind kept drifting back to the three main trainers who had become such an integral part of my routine. —Avijit, Subhas, and Harinder. Over time, they had become more than just instructors at the gym; they were guiding forces, shaping not just my body but my approach to life.

I could still feel the electric energy of the gym whenever Avijit was around. His infectious enthusiasm was impossible to ignore. He didn't just lead workouts; he elevated them. His passion for fitness radiated through the room, igniting something in everyone, no matter how tired or unmotivated they were when they arrived. Avijit's energy was magnetic—it pulled you in, pushed you harder, and left you feeling more capable than when you started.

Then there was Subhas, with his methodical approach to every session. Where Avijit was all about energy, Subhas was about precision. He had a way of breaking down even the most complex movements into digestible steps. His approach made fitness feel accessible, even to beginners, as if he could guide anyone through the toughest of workouts. He wasn't just a trainer; he was a strategist, someone who taught us how to master each move by focusing on the fundamentals. His attention to detail made me realise that fitness wasn't just about strength—it was about technique, discipline, and understanding your own body.

Harinder, the quiet force in the gym, was a different kind of presence altogether. He didn't speak much, but when he did, it carried weight. His calm demeanour acted as an anchor during the most gruelling workouts. There was something deeply reassuring about his steady gaze and his subtle nods of encouragement. He made me feel that no matter how tough things got, I could push through. Harinder represented quiet resilience—strength in stillness, perseverance in silence.

The impact of these three trainers extended far beyond the physical space of the gym. They were, in every sense, role models of accountability and consistency. They didn't just talk about discipline; they embodied it. Day after day, they showed up with the same level of dedication, focus, and passion, regardless of what was happening in their personal lives. It was their actions, more than their words, that instilled in me a deep understanding of what it means to be consistent.

As I progressed through the warm-up, I reflected on how much their presence had shaped my perspective on fitness and, in turn, life. Consistency wasn't just about showing up to the gym; it was about showing up for yourself, for your goals, for your commitments—every single day, even when it was hard, even when you didn't feel like it. The physical workouts became a metaphor for something bigger. They taught me that real progress comes not from grand efforts but from the small, consistent actions we take day in and day out.

In the beginning, I thought of fitness as purely physical. It was about sculpting my body, losing weight, and becoming stronger. But as time went on, I realised that the lessons I was learning in the gym had far-reaching effects. The discipline I was developing in my workouts began to seep into other areas of my life—my work, my relationships, my personal goals. I started to apply the same principles of consistency and accountability that I learned from the trainers to everything I did. And with that, my life began to change in ways I hadn't anticipated.

But it wasn't always easy. There were days when the weight of the world felt too heavy to bear, when the thought of dragging myself out of bed at 4:15 a.m. seemed impossible. Those were the days when I questioned my own strength, both mentally and physically. Yet, on those days, I would think of Avijit's energy, Subhas's methodical guidance, and Harinder's quiet encouragement. Their commitment fuelled mine. It reminded me that showing up, especially on the hard days, was what made the difference. It was easy to work hard when everything was going well, but true growth came from pushing through when everything felt difficult.

Over time, something shifted within me. My journey wasn't about reaching the final destination anymore—it was about embracing the process. It was about growing a little every day, about showing up and putting in the work even when I didn't feel like it. Slowly, this mindset began to extend beyond the gym. Whether it was tackling a difficult project at work or nurturing important relationships, I realised that the same principles applied: consistency, effort, patience.

As the weeks turned into months, I began to see the changes—not just in my body, but in my mind. I was more disciplined, more focused, more determined. The lessons I had learned from my trainers about accountability, discipline, and consistency had become part of who I was. What had started as a fitness goal had transformed into a life philosophy. Consistency wasn't just about fitness anymore; it had become the key to unlocking success in every area of my life.

Looking back, I realised that the moments that shaped me weren't the big, dramatic milestones. It wasn't the days when I hit a new personal record or the times when everything went perfectly. The real transformation happened in the small, daily choices—the decision to get up early, the choice to push through one more set, the commitment to show up when it would have been easier to stay home. It was those small, seemingly insignificant moments that added up over time to create real, lasting change.

The trainers had laid the groundwork, but ultimately, it was my responsibility to build upon it. They had shown me that consistency wasn't just a tool for fitness—it was the key to success in everything. And as I embraced that lesson, I found myself moving closer to becoming the person I had always wanted to be.

Through the ups and downs of this journey, I've come to understand that there's no final goal, no ultimate destination where everything falls into place. The real value lies in the process—in the act of showing up, day after day, and putting in the work. The workouts have become a metaphor for life itself. There will always be challenges, moments of doubt, and times when the path forward seems unclear.

But if I've learned anything from Avijit, Subhas, and Harinder, it's that the key to success lies in *consistency*. Consistency has woven itself into the fabric of my life like an invisible thread, binding my efforts and my journey together. It's a quiet force, steadfast and unpretentious, driving my progress day after day. There's nothing glamorous about it; no flashiness or dramatic overnight transformations. It's about a steady, unwavering commitment to the process. And through this, I've come to understand that true strength lies not in grand gestures but in the quiet persistence of showing up, even when the motivation wanes.

As I continued on my path of consistency, I uncovered a crucial truth: improvement isn't just about sticking to a routine—it's about the interplay of strength and balance. These elements aren't isolated; they're interconnected aspects of the same journey.

Gravity's Challenge: The Balance Breakthrough

Several months went by, and I was truly getting into the rhythm of being a Fit Buddy when someone in my group mentioned TRX. It sounded fascinating and exciting, so, on June 16, 2023, I finally decided to take the plunge and try it out.

What really gets my adrenaline pumping on Fridays isn't just the end of the workweek—it's the thrill of the TRX session ahead. The real excitement starts days before the class, as I eagerly anticipate securing a spot. My phone becomes a relentless reminder, buzzing with notifications that urge me to grab my slot before they disappear. This seemingly ordinary task turns into a high-stakes race against time, and I tackle it with a competitive zeal that would make anyone proud. The whole process feels almost cinematic, and when I finally snag my place, it's like winning a victory as the slots fill up one by one.

For those unfamiliar with TRX (Total Resistance eXercises), let me offer a glimpse into its fascinating world. Imagine a fitness approach that blends versatility with transformative potential—a method that challenges both body and mind. Some may already be familiar with TRX, while others might view it as one of the industry's best-kept secrets. Either way, TRX represents a profound exploration into strength, balance, and the invaluable life lessons that extend far beyond a typical workout routine.

The origins of TRX trace back to Randy Hetrick, a former U.S. Navy SEAL whose resourcefulness and inventive spirit gave birth to this revolutionary suspension training system. Hetrick's background in military training and problem-solving led him to create a fitness tool that has since redefined the way we approach exercise. What began as a practical solution for maintaining fitness in confined spaces has evolved into a global fitness phenomenon. The TRX system, comprising straps and handles, facilitates a diverse array of bodyweight exercises. This ingenious setup enables a dynamic workout that engages multiple muscle groups simultaneously, making it a game-changer in the fitness world. Each session becomes a comprehensive experience, tailored to individual goals and needs.

At our Fitness Centre, TRX has transcended its role as just another workout. It has become the heartbeat of our fitness routine, a cornerstone that binds us together. What began as an intriguing exercise modality has transformed into a cherished weekly ritual. This ritual unites our eclectic group of fitness enthusiasts—Aashna, Shalini, Malini, Anand, Mahesh, Sudhakar, and me—into a community bound by shared experiences and mutual respect. The practice has woven itself into the fabric of our lives, becoming a source of memorable moments and a profound sense of camaraderie.

The weekly ritual begins with the opening of TRX booking slots, a moment charged with anticipation and excitement. The process of securing a spot feels akin to grabbing tickets for a much-anticipated concert. As soon as the booking window opens, we all scramble with a sense of urgency, eager to claim our places before they disappear. The competition is fierce, the excitement palpable. Securing a spot is not merely about claiming a place in the class; it's about earning our ticket to a communal experience that promises both challenge and triumph.

My weekly TRX sessions have evolved into more than just exercise. It has become a testament to my collective commitment and passion for fitness. The anticipation that accompanies the booking process is matched only by the thrill of the sessions themselves. As I, along with other members gather each week, the energy in the room is electric. I approach the TRX straps not just as pieces of equipment but as instruments that would unite me in my pursuit of strength, balance, and personal growth.

Among the members, Malini adds a unique and endearing flavour to our TRX sessions. Her slightly mischievous habit of occasionally missing her booked slot has become a cherished part of our group dynamic. It's a running joke that never fails to elicit laughter and camaraderie. Despite her hit-or-miss attendance, Malini's infectious enthusiasm and lively spirit are integral to our sessions. Her presence—or absence—always sparks a sense of humor and keeps the atmosphere light and enjoyable.

My initial encounter with TRX was nothing short of an adventure. The system's design seemed to promise a dynamic experience, something that could be as fun and exhilarating as a circus act. Imagine performing stunts that defy gravity, balancing on the edge of your limits, and feeling like you're part of a performance that's both thrilling and demanding.

The TRX setup, with its straps and handles, appeared almost playful in its complexity. It looks like a piece of gym equipment that had stepped out of a whimsical imagination, inviting you to twist, turn, and stretch in ways that seemed more akin to a dance or acrobatics than a traditional workout. I was curious, intrigued by the sight of these tools and the promise they held. It was like seeing a new form of entertainment—something that would challenge not only my body but also my mind.

As I continued my journey with TRX (Total Resistance eXercises), the playful veneer I initially saw began to peel away, revealing a far more intense and demanding reality. What once seemed like a fun game transformed into a rigorous test of strength and balance. The initial allure of TRX, with its straps and handles that appeared inviting and straightforward, soon revealed its true nature—a challenging workout that required a deeper commitment than I had anticipated.

Every TRX session starts with an internal struggle that feels like a subplot in my own personal sitcom. The dialogue in my head is a familiar one: "I could be lounging on the couch right now, binge-watching cat videos, comfortably ensconced in my blanket." Yet, despite the seductive temptation of relaxation and the cozy whispers from my bed, I am compelled to uphold the art of discipline. This commitment transforms me from a 'weekend warrior' into a 'weekday champion' proving that dedication to fitness is not confined to weekends but is a continuous, everyday commitment.

Let me paint you a picture of what this dedication looks like. Picture a dynamic lunge with my foot strapped into a TRX strap. It feels akin to performing an intricate ballet move while someone else is holding your foot and you're fervently hoping that gravity won't play tricks on you. The exercise demands a delicate balance and a combination of strength and coordination, requiring both physical prowess and mental focus. Or consider the suspended push-up, where I'm hanging mid-air, challenging the basic laws of physics and my instinct for self-preservation. Each movement pushes my limits in ways I had not anticipated, compelling me to adapt and persevere while striving to maintain a semblance of grace.

Through these intense and demanding experiences, I've come to understand that TRX is more than just a series of stretches or physical exertion. It is a profound exercise in adapting my body to new positions while striving to maintain balance and grace. It's not just about avoiding a face-first collision with the floor; it's about embracing the challenge of pushing beyond my limits and emerging stronger on the other side.

The true beauty of TRX lies in its emphasis on incremental progress. As I push through each session, my mind navigates two critical aspects: endurance and confidence. Endurance in TRX training is a beast of its own, involving not just physical exertion but also a mental game where I might feel on the brink of collapse, all while meeting the relentless demands of reps and sets. It's like running a marathon with a bag of bricks—except these bricks are my self-doubt, and the marathon is an endless series of challenges. I realised that the key to mastering endurance lies in embracing the discomfort, greeting it with a determined grin and a grunt, and pushing through despite the overwhelming urge to quit.

Achieving balance within the realm of TRX training is a sophisticated ballet of core strength, coordination, and focus. My core muscles work like undercover operatives, ensuring my stability and keeping me upright. They perform their duties silently but effectively, making sure I don't topple over or lose my footing, even when I'm pushing my limits. Coordination steps into the spotlight, acting as the ringmaster of this intricate circus. It orchestrates the synchronised movement of every limb, ensuring that each exercise is performed with precision and grace. Without it, the complex choreography of TRX training would devolve into a chaotic display of flailing limbs and missed steps.

Focus serves as the vigilant spotter, always watchful and ready to intervene. It prevents me from straying off course, avoiding a dreaded face-plant that could easily make its way into the blooper reel of my workout sessions. This mental acuity ensures I remain on track, balancing carefully and executing each movement with intention and control. The interplay of these elements—core strength, coordination, and focus—is crucial in the TRX training process, creating a harmonious and effective workout experience.

Navigating the complexities of TRX training involves surmounting a series of challenges, each contributing to a profound sense of achievement. Every demanding workout completed, and every new skill acquired, fosters a deep well of self-respect and pride. This ongoing process of small victories—achieving just a little more today than yesterday—bolsters my confidence, not only within the confines of the gym but also in other areas of my life. The steady progression from one milestone to the next reinforces my belief in my abilities, proving that I am capable of overcoming obstacles and achieving my goals.

Through TRX training, I have learned that true STRENGTH and BALANCE extend beyond mere physical attributes. They encompass a broader spectrum of mental and emotional dimensions. Facing challenges head-on, enduring discomfort, and celebrating the incremental victories that punctuate the journey are integral components of both fitness and personal growth. This holistic approach demonstrates that the path to greater strength and balance is not a one-dimensional pursuit. Instead, it is a multifaceted endeavour that weaves together physical prowess, mental resilience, and emotional fortitude.

Reflecting on my journey through TRX training, it becomes clear that the lessons learned extend far beyond the gym. The experience has taught me that achieving balance and strength requires a balance of mind and body, a delicate interplay of physical, mental, and emotional elements. Each workout, each challenge overcome, contributes to a greater understanding of what it means to be truly strong and balanced.

Flex It Like a Yogi: Unveiling the Power of Stretching

Aug 7, 2023. I strolled into the Fitness Centre, a gleaming shrine of steel and sweat, fully prepared to dive headfirst into the world of strength training, boxing, and the occasional treadmill - fuelled existential crisis. My eyes lit up with excitement—the weights, the punching bags, and the limitless possibilities spread out before me like a playground for grown-ups. I was like a kid in a candy store, except instead of sugary treats, I craved dumbbells and heavy lifts.

Yoga? That was just a distant thought—more like a soft, zen-like whisper lingering in the background, gently reminding me of flexibility. It wasn't loud or flashy, not like the adrenaline-pumping allure of lifting or boxing, but more like a librarian quietly slipping a book into my hand, subtle and persistent, nudging me toward a path I wasn't quite ready to embrace.

"Hey there," it seemed to say, *"Why don't you give me a try?"*

I looked at Yoga as one might regard an unexpected guest at a wild party—confused, slightly suspicious, but polite enough to offer a drink. And so began my less-than-illustrious romance with Yoga. Imagine me, awkwardly stumbling through poses like a giraffe attempting ballet on roller skates. There I was, twisting and bending with all the elegance of a pretzel in a wind tunnel.

My first attempts at Yoga felt less like a serene dance and more like a series of unfortunate events, each one culminating in a graceful collapse onto the mat, staring blankly at the ceiling.

I pondered whether my body was secretly designed for something less... bendy. Maybe, just maybe, my genes were telling me that Yoga was a cruel joke played by the universe. Yet, amidst the tumbleweeds of my attempts, there were those small victories—the fleeting moments when I managed to hold a pose for an extra second without toppling over. These tiny triumphs were like little nuggets of gold in my otherwise clumsy treasure hunt. It wasn't love at first stretch. No, indeed. My relationship with Yoga was more akin to a slow, awkward dance, where each misstep brought us closer together. Each session was a step towards acceptance, like learning to appreciate a song you initially thought was utterly annoying. Despite the wobbles, the occasional face-plant, and the constant internal debates about whether I should just stick to lifting weights, Yoga began to chip away at my reluctance.

Slowly but surely, Yoga's subtle charm won me over. It wasn't the grand, sweeping gestures of romance but rather the gentle persistence that drew me in. I found myself looking forward to the sessions, enjoying the odd sense of accomplishment when I managed to hold a pose without resembling a malfunctioning robot. Yoga transitioned from being a reluctant fling to a steadfast companion in my fitness journey.

So here's the lesson: If I could hang in there and manage to stay on the mat, perhaps there was hope for me. Yoga, with its gentle nudges and quirky poses, turned from a dreaded challenge into a beloved part of my routine. It proved that sometimes the best things come from stepping out of your comfort zone, even if it means occasionally toppling over like a poorly balanced Jenga Tower.

In Yoga, having a well-trained instructor makes all the difference, and thankfully, our Fitness Centre delivers just that. But what really makes a Yoga instructor special? It's not just about reciting pose names that sound like they belong to a Harry

Potter's spell book. It's about creating an environment where Yoga feels approachable for everyone—whether an individual is a seasoned yogi or someone who still wonders if 'downward dog' might be the title of the latest Netflix binge!

Enter Harinder, my Yoga wizard at the Fitness Centre. Harinder doesn't just lead a class; he transforms it into an epic adventure. He takes the most complex asanas—those poses with names that could be straight out of a fantasy novel—and breaks them down into manageable pieces. It's like having a GPS for your body, guiding you through the labyrinth of limbs with a touch of humour.

Picture this: You're in the middle of a pose, feeling zen and ready to congratulate yourself on your near-perfect execution when Harinder swoops in like a fitness fairy godparent. With a gentle nudge or a kind correction, he turns your "*Close enough...*" into "*Nailed it*!" It's like magic—minus the sparkles.

Harinder's hands-on approach is where the real enchantment happens. He's not just observing from a distance like a Yoga sage on a mountaintop; he's right there, adjusting my posture with the precision of a sculptor chiselling marble. He ensures every twist and turn is just right, turning your Yoga practice from a mere attempt into a masterpiece. The best part? Harinder makes even the most complicated poses feel like a fun challenge rather than a gruelling test of willpower. With him, I'm not just trying to stretch into a pretzel shape; I'm embarking on a journey where every adjustment brings me closer to Yoga greatness. In his class, Yoga isn't just about bending and stretching; it's about having fun while doing it. It's about that feeling of triumph when I finally master a pose you once thought was impossible. It's about the laughter shared over a particularly tricky asana and the satisfaction of knowing that I'm not just improving my flexibility but also enjoying every moment of the process. The rhythm of Harinder's classes is magical. He makes the hour fly by, as if I enter in a fitness time warp.

But don't be fooled by his serene, almost angelic demeanour. Harinder has a mischievous streak that can make even the most dedicated yogi question their life choices. Take his counting, for example. What should have been a simple numerical progression becomes a test of endurance that makes a marathon look like a stroll in the park. Imagine holding a pose, sweat pouring down, muscles trembling, and Harinder chanting, *"1…2…3…4…5…6…7…8…9…"* while you beg for that elusive *"10!"* which seems to be hiding in a distant galaxy. When he finally says that gloriously elusive *"10!"* the members collapse into fits of giggles and high-fives, celebrating tiny victories that only fellow yogis can truly appreciate.

In his group classes, I learnt that the journey is not just about mastering the perfect pose or achieving personal bests. It's about embracing the communal struggle, finding joy in the shared experience, and surviving together with a smile (and maybe a few strategically placed ice packs). The beauty of it all is that, in the end, I'm not just a part of the sweaty bunch, stretching enthusiasts; I also represent a tight-knit crew of camaraderie, bound together by shared pain and collective triumphs.

Just when I thought I had Yoga all figured out, our Fitness Centre threw me a curveball—enter "Evolve Yoga," the new twist (and yes, quite literally) on the practice.

Picture this: Yoga with circular props that made us feel like we were auditioning for the role of a human carousel. It was like taking a perfectly good video game and adding a new, ridiculously tricky level—complete with unexpected plot twists and quirky obstacles.

But fear not! Harinder, our Yoga maestro, was not just unfazed but positively thrilled by this new challenge. With the grace of a ballet dancer and the patience of a saint, he guided me through this new dimension of Yoga like he was leading me on a magical journey through a land of rolling circles and swirling movements. His expertise turned what could have been a chaotic mess into a fluid dance of flexibility and balance.

The introduction of these circular props was like Yoga's version of a plot twist. Suddenly, what was once straightforward became a thrilling adventure. I was no longer just stretching and bending; I was navigating a new world where my mat was rolling in circles, and my poses had to adapt to this new reality. It was a bit like trying to play hopscotch on a trampoline—exciting, a little confusing, and immensely fun.

These circular structures didn't just add complexity; they brought a whole new layer of engagement to my practice. It was a vivid reminder that Yoga, much like life, is in constant flux. Just when I thought I've got it all down, there's always a new way to challenge myself. The circles weren't just fancy props; they were metaphors for the endless cycle of effort, progress, and those little stumbles that make the journey all the more interesting.

As my Yoga journey rolled on, something magical happened—I went from being the clumsy newbie who couldn't touch his toes to a full-blown Yoga enthusiast, basking in the glow of my newfound flexibility! Gone were the days of awkwardly flopping onto my mat and questioning if my body was secretly made of bricks. Instead, I found myself thriving in a Yoga community that cheered for every small victory, celebrated each pose I conquered, and revelled in every little bit of progress.

Yoga, which once seemed like a daunting challenge and a source of endless anxiety, had transformed into my personal sanctuary. It became my cozy retreat, my go-to haven for unwinding, and, unexpectedly, a fountain of joy. Who knew that contorting into poses that initially seemed impossible could turn into moments of triumph and bliss?

Every class felt like a mini-celebration, with my fellow yogis and I high-fiving each other for mastering a tricky pose or simply for showing up with a smile. It was as if, I was a part of a giant, stretchy, and infinitely supportive Yoga family, cheering my fellow yogis on through every bend and twist. From struggling to touch my toes to feeling like a Yoga superstar, my journey was filled with unexpected joy and delightful surprises. Yoga had gone from being a reluctant challenge to an exhilarating adventure, reminding me that sometimes, the best things in life come when you least expect them.

The once-reluctant yogi, now thriving on the mat, decides to take the plunge into the wider world of fitness. You'd think it would be a serious business, right? Think again! Fitness is about more than just sweating buckets; it's about embracing the journey with a big grin and a side of fun. This isn't about competing to be the best; it's about coming together to have a blast while getting stronger and healthier. Every fitness session becomes an opportunity to bond with like-minded individuals, to cheer each other on, and to create memories that go beyond the gym.

Sneaker Trap: How One Wrong Choice Left Me Limping

I'm the kind of guy who shows up for his workouts on time, ready to tackle the next challenge. The gym is my sanctuary, a place where I can disconnect from the outside world and focus on my body's needs. Whether it's a strength training circuit or a cardio blast, I'm all in, pushing myself with each rep and breath. But on this particular day, things went south – all because of a simple yet costly mistake: wearing the wrong shoes!

It was Aug 30, 2023. It started like any other gym day. I grabbed my gym bag, filled my water bottle, and laced up my shoes. Only today, instead of my usual trainers, I made the rookie mistake of slipping on an old pair of sneakers. They looked fine, I had spent a good amount of money in owning them – barely worn and comfortable, but there was a reason I'd stopped using them for workouts. I had forgotten that they weren't designed for intense gym sessions, especially the kind that involved a lot of jumping, like today's workout.

But hey, a shoe's a shoe, right? Wrong.

The warm-up went well enough. A couple of stretches, some light jogging in place, a few squats to get the blood flowing. Then came the real deal: high-intensity interval training (HIIT), filled with all kinds of jumping exercises – box jumps, burpees, and, of course, the notorious jumping jacks. I hadn't anticipated what was about to happen.

With each jump, I could feel my toes jamming against the front of my sneakers. But I ignored it, convinced it was just a little discomfort that would pass once my body got into the rhythm of the workout. As the session progressed, though, the discomfort turned into something more painful — a sharp, stabbing sensation in my big toe. By the time we reached the last round of burpees, my foot was throbbing, but still, I pushed through, stubborn as ever.

When the workout ended, I peeled off my shoes and socks to check the damage. My big toe was red, swollen, and hot to the touch. What was supposed to be an invigorating workout had turned into an unexpected lesson in the importance of proper footwear. I could feel the throbbing with each step I took. Toe inflammation? Over a pair of shoes? This was a new low.

As I sat there massaging my sore foot, my trainer walked over and took one look at my shoes, shaking his head. *"Looks like those shoes have lost their mojo, huh?"* he said with a hint of sympathy. I nodded, feeling a bit sheepish. Then he explained something I really should have known: just like you wouldn't use a hammer to screw in a nail, you can't use the wrong shoes for a high-impact workout like this.

After that conversation with my trainer, I decided to dig deeper into the importance of footwear. The more I read, the more it became clear that the right shoes are essential—especially for high-impact exercises like jumping jacks, burpees, and box jumps. I used to think shoes were all about comfort or style, but they're so much more than that. They're your primary defence against injury, offering the support and cushioning your body needs to absorb the stress of intense movements.

Every time I jump or land, the impact needs to be absorbed somewhere, and without the right footwear, that force goes directly to the joints, muscles, and feet. The old pair I had thrown on that day simply wasn't up to the challenge. Lacking adequate support, my feet had slid inside the shoes, causing friction with every move. That friction, in turn, led to swelling and inflammation in my toes.

As painful as my experience was, I quickly discovered I wasn't alone. Over the next few weeks, I heard similar stories from others at the gym. Suresh, one of my workout buddies, had made the same mistake, wearing his old running shoes to a weightlifting session. Without the necessary support, he ended up with a twisted ankle.

Fenny, another regular, had worn minimalist shoes—those thin-soled barefoot shoes—for a plyometric workout. Halfway through the session, she felt a sharp pain in her heel. The next morning, she was limping, and later found out she had developed plantar fasciitis. Like me, she learned the hard way that the wrong footwear can cause serious damage.

The message was loud and clear: wearing the wrong shoes can lead to a cascade of problems, from minor aches to major injuries like stress fractures, tendonitis, and plantar fasciitis. Worse still, injuries can sideline anyone from the workouts we love for weeks, even months.

In my case, the swelling in my toes was caused by the repetitive stress placed on my feet. Every time I jumped, my body weight came crashing down, and without the right shoes to absorb that shock, my feet took the brunt of it. Over time, this constant impact led to inflammation in the muscles and joints of my feet, particularly in my toes.

The constant friction between my toes and the inside of the shoe aggravated the soft tissues, leading to even more inflammation. My body's natural response to this irritation was to send extra fluid to the area, causing swelling, or edema. It was a painful reminder of just how important the right equipment—especially shoes—can be in preventing injury.

After a few days of rest and some anti-inflammatory treatments, the swelling finally subsided. But the lesson stayed with me. I'd always known that shoes were important, but I hadn't fully understood just how critical they are, especially for high-impact workouts. Now, every time I lace up, I'm reminded of that painful day.

I invested in a quality pair of cross-training shoes—designed specifically for the types of exercises I love to do—and they've made all the difference. The right shoes provide the cushioning, support, and stability I need to keep my body safe while pushing myself in the gym.

If there's one key takeaway from my experience, it's that not all shoes are created equal. Just because a pair of shoes works for walking or running doesn't mean they're suitable for weightlifting, jumping, or any other high-intensity workout. Each type of exercise places different demands on your feet, and it's crucial to choose footwear that's designed to meet those demands.

For jumping exercises, like the ones that caused my injury, cross-training shoes are ideal. They provide the right mix of stability and cushioning, allowing the feet to absorb the impact without putting undue stress on your joints and muscles. Running shoes, while great for forward motion, don't offer the lateral support or structure necessary for workouts involving a lot of jumping or sudden changes in direction.

One painful experience ended up being a hidden blessing. It gave me a newfound appreciation for the crucial role footwear plays in fitness. Now, each time I step into the gym, I pause to recognise that my shoes do more than just keep my feet comfortable—they shield me from injury, enable me to push myself harder, and aid in quicker recovery. I've also become vigilant about watching for signs that it's time to invest in a new pair of high-quality gym shoes before my current ones lose their effectiveness.

As I learned the hard way, wearing the wrong shoes can leave me limping out of the gym, taking me away from the workouts I love and plunging me into weeks, or even months, of painful recovery.

Phase II

BEING A FIT CHAMP

Becoming a Fit Champ from a Fit Buddy comes with its own share of responsibilities. As a Fit Buddy, the journey was all about learning, growing, and finding my place within the fitness community. But transitioning into a Fit Champ adds a whole new layer of meaning—one where I'm not just focused on my own fitness goals, but also on supporting and inspiring others.

A Fit Champ is someone who embodies the spirit of leadership, motivation, and community, guiding newcomers and helping them navigate their own fitness journeys. It's a role that demands not just physical strength, but also emotional intelligence and a willingness to lift others as much as you lift weights.

A Fit Champ is someone who has transitioned from being a learner to a leader, embracing the responsibility of setting an example for others. It's about showing up consistently, not just for personal progress, but also for the sake of the fitness community. In many ways, it's like being the lead actor in a motivational movie where the script revolves around commitment, perseverance, and mutual encouragement. Each day brings new opportunities to lift others, whether by demonstrating the right way to perform a workout or simply offering words of encouragement during a tough session.

The role of a Fit Champ isn't just about showing up at the gym—it's about fostering a supportive environment where everyone feels encouraged. Whether it's leading by example or cracking a joke to ease someone's nerves, I've learned that guiding newcomers is as much about empathy as it is about fitness techniques. This responsibility has honed my leadership skills, teaching me valuable lessons in communication, motivation, and teamwork that extend far beyond the gym. Whether I'm at work or navigating personal relationships, the skills I've developed as a Fit Champ are applicable in every facet of life.

But being a Fit Champ isn't just about responsibility—it's about having fun. Watching someone go from being intimidated by the gym to thriving in their workouts is incredibly rewarding. It's like being part of a real-life success story, where every chapter is filled with perseverance, progress, and a whole lot of joy. As I guide others, I get to witness firsthand the incredible transformations, reminding me of the power of fitness and community.

The journey from Fit Buddy to Fit Champ has been enthralling, both personally and professionally. It's shown me that fitness is more than just exercise—it's about connection, growth, and shared triumphs.

In the following chapters, I'll walk you through my later and present days (Phase II) i.e being a Fit Champ. Here you will witness how the transition from Fit Buddy to Fit Champ not only transforms individuals but also creates a thriving fitness community. These stories will inspire you to embrace fitness, not just as a solitary pursuit, but as an adventure that's best enjoyed together.

Building Bonds and Breaking Sweat: Embracing Camaraderie at our Fitness Centre

It was Sep 13, 2023 and exactly at 4.45 am, that obnoxious alarm was at it again...

BEEP! BEEP!! BEEP!!!

I was dragged out of dreamland. Who in their right mind is up at this hour? Oh right, I am. Because I've willingly signed up for this madness called the 5:30 a.m. workout at our Fitness Centre. If there's one thing I've learned from this early morning routine, it's that the first victory of the day is simply rolling out of bed.

By 5:15 a.m., the city of Bengaluru is still rubbing the sleep from its eyes, but not at our Fitness Centre. Here, the air buzzes with the kind of energy that only comes from a mix of adrenaline, caffeine, and sheer willpower. The regulars start trickling in, each with their own brand of enthusiasm - some cheerful, some still half-asleep but trying to fake it. And then there's Malini, our ever-smiling, ever-ready fitness warrior. Malini arrives at 5:20 a.m. sharp, ready to take on the world—or at least her morning workout. She steps into her designated square on the gym floor, which, let's be honest, feels a bit like docking into a spaceship.

"Prepare for launch," she thinks, as she takes in the sea of familiar faces. This grid is her sanctuary, where she's about to battle the forces of gravity, calories, and yesterday's cheat meal.

With 5:27 a.m. on the clock, the scene is set. It's the calm before the storm, and I can almost hear the collective gulp as everyone braces themselves for what's to come. There's a comforting hum of whispered "Good Mornings" and a few groggy nods exchanged across the room. Malini catches sight of a familiar smirk across the way – a fellow early bird who's just as committed, or perhaps as crazy, as she is. Her inner monologue kicks in: *"Well, at least I've got someone to share my pain with!"*

At precisely 5:30 a.m., the trainer steps up with the kind of punctuality that could put a Swiss watch to shame. The music starts, the warm-up begins, and the grid of fitness warriors spring to life in perfect synchrony—well, almost.

Warm-ups at our Fitness Centre are a unique blend of dynamic stretches and synchronised movements that are supposed to prepare us for the workout ahead. But let's be real, it's also a chance to see if our body still functions at this ungodly hour. Malini has mastered the art of pretending she knows what she's doing, stealing glances at the others to make sure she's not alone in her early morning awkwardness.

As she navigates through the stretches, she notices the usual suspects in the room. There's the '*Flex Guru,*' Anish, who never misses a chance to show off his impeccable form; the '*Overachiever,*' Pratham who's already halfway through the workout in the warm-up; and the '*Newbie,*' Shraddha who looks like she's reconsidering every life choice that led them here. And then there's Malini's personal favourite: '*The Talker,*' Varun who somehow manages to carry on a full-blown conversation while the rest of them are just trying to breathe.

But it's all in good fun. Because at our Fitness Centre, no one is left behind. If I trip, stumble, or get lost in the routine, there's always a friendly hand (or a cheeky comment) to pull me back on track. Malini can't help but grin as she catches a wink from *'The Talker'*, who is apparently mid-sentence and mid-burpee at the same time.

"How does he do that?" Malini wonders. "Maybe that's his superpower."

Now, the real fun begins. For the next 50 minutes, this room transforms into a battleground of grit, sweat, and a surprising amount of laughter. The class is a whirlwind of high-fives, groans, and the occasional *"Did I really sign up for this?"* moments. Malini is in her element, thriving off the collective energy that turns this workout into a kind of group therapy session—with squats.

At our Fitness Centre, workouts are more than just a physical challenge; they're a mental and emotional release. Whether I'm frustrated from work, stressed about life, or just need to burn off the weekend's indulgences, there's something cathartic about pushing myself alongside others who are right there with me. And the best part? No one takes themselves too seriously.

During the circuit training, there's a friendly competition brewing between the workout buddies. Each pair tries to outdo the other in reps, form, or just sheer determination. Malini pairs up with the *'Overachiever'*, knowing full well that he'll push her limits—and secretly hoping she'll make him break a sweat. Meanwhile, the *'Talker'* is still chatting away, now with the *'Flex Guru'*, who seems genuinely impressed with his ability to multitask. As the minutes tick by, the camaraderie only grows stronger. Malini's group rallies together, encouraging each other to keep going when the burn sets in. They swap motivational quotes, inside jokes, and the occasional dramatic eye roll when the trainer introduces yet another round of burpees. The air is thick with effort and the faint scent of *"Why am I doing this to myself?"* But despite the groans, there's a sense of collective accomplishment that keeps everyone going.

By the time the clock strikes 6:20 a.m., the class is nearing its end, and I'd think the intensity would start to wane. But no, this is our Fitness Centre, where the final moments are just as crucial as the first. The session wraps up with a cool-down and a group stretch that feels more like a victory lap than a chore.

And then, it's time for the grand finale: the *"Pic of the Day."* This isn't just any photo. It's a badge of honour, proof that you survived yet another round of early morning torture with a smile (or at least a grimace). The class gathers around, sweaty but triumphant, and strikes a pose that screams, *"Rise and Shine!"* Malini finds her spot in the front, next to the *'Flex Guru'* and the *'Talker'*, who—surprise, surprise—is still mid-sentence. As the camera clicks, there's a collective sense of pride that washes over the group. We did it. Together. And tomorrow, we'll do it all over again. But for now, it's time to grab that much-needed post-workout smoothie and bask in the glow of a morning well spent.

As the workout draws to a close, the group, drenched in sweat and still riding the adrenaline wave, eagerly anticipates the next big thing—a refreshing shower, maybe, or perhaps just collapsing onto a nearby bench. But today, fate has something far more entertaining in store.

Enter Mahesh, striding into the holding area with the kind of swagger usually reserved for rock stars or the guy who just aced the office presentation. The air crackles with excitement, the kind you'd expect if someone walked in holding a box of fresh, hot pizza. But Mahesh has something even better—cucumbers!

With a dramatic flourish, Mahesh unveils his green treasures, presenting them like a magician revealing his final, mind-blowing trick. It's as if he's saying, *"You thought I was just another guy with a post-workout glow? Think again!"*

The room erupts into a symphony of astonished gasps and appreciative cheers, as if he'd just pulled off the most daring heist of the century. Sudhakar, always quick with a quip, doesn't miss a beat. *"Oh look, it's the Great Cucumber Caper!"* he declares, his voice dripping with mock grandeur. The group bursts into laughter, the kind that bubbles up from deep within, fuelled by the sheer absurdity of the moment. As Mahesh continues to distribute his crunchy loot, Sudhakar isn't done with his witty commentary. *"I can smell burning rubber,"* he adds with a grin, *"So we must have a new hero in town!"* The statement hangs in the air for a moment, before the group collectively agrees that Mahesh has earned a new title. And so, in the blink of an eye and with a unanimous vote, Mahesh is dubbed *'Krishna'*. The title comes with all the pomp and circumstance one might expect, including an imaginary cucumber-themed crown that Sudhakar insists Mahesh now wears at all times.

The cucumbers themselves are met with sheer delight, as if they're the most decadent of treats. Who knew a humble veggie could inspire such joy? As Mahesh hands out slices with the enthusiasm of a food critic recommending the day's special, it's clear that he's basking in the glory of his new role. His smile is practically glowing, brighter than the morning Sun that's just beginning to peek through the clouds. Each slice is received with the reverence usually reserved for a sacred offering, and the group savours the crisp, cool refreshment like a rare delicacy.

Meanwhile, Malini, ever the enthusiastic supporter of all things ridiculous, has already decided that this moment needs a proper tribute. Without missing a beat, she launches into an off-key karaoke rendition of *"Hail to the Cucumber King,"* her voice wobbling through the notes with more enthusiasm than accuracy. The group joins in, some more reluctantly than others, but all with grins plastered across their faces. Mahesh, now fully embracing his role as *'Krishna'*, graciously accepts the honour, nodding along as if he's always known this day would come.

As the impromptu celebration continues, the group can't help but marvel at how the morning has unfolded. What started as just another workout session has transformed into something infinitely more memorable, thanks to Mahesh and his unexpected offering. The CAMARADERIE in the room is palpable, a reminder that sometimes, it's the simplest things—a shared laugh, a surprising twist—that bring people closer together. The cucumbers, once just a post-workout snack, have become the symbol of the day's shared joy, and Mahesh, the unlikeliest of heroes, has solidified his place in the group's lore.

Aashna and Promila, the wise sages of the fitness realm, often remind everyone of an essential truth: *"Fitness routines should never grow monotonous; there's always so much fun to look forward to at 5.30 a.m."* And they're right. The 5.30 a.m. workouts are like a daily adventure where the treasure is good health, and the map is drawn with the chalk of camaraderie.

Then there's Prateek, the motorcycle maverick. He rides his KTM motorbike a mere 500 meters from his home to the Fitness Centre. But here's the kicker—he takes the long route on the way back. Why? Because apparently, a short ride isn't enough to celebrate surviving the morning workout. Prateek's level-headedness and friendly demeanour make him a marvel in class. He's the kind of guy who makes everyone wonder if he's secretly sipping on a magic elixir of calm and coolness.

Speaking of marvels, let's talk about Vinita, our yoga aficionado. In Yoga class, Vinita is the unsung hero who aids the trainer in counting down those last agonising seconds of the plank. With her unwavering support, the final count of *"10"* becomes less of a struggle and more of a celebratory milestone. Vinita's timing is impeccable, and her presence is a reminder that even in the toughest moments, there's always a helping hand—or a precise count.

Let's not forget Nanda, Aanchal, and Reema, whose enthusiasm and inspiration keep the group bubbling with energy. These are the folks who bring the kind of excitement that makes you look forward to the next workout as if it's a season finale of your favourite show.

And speaking of excitement, there's a legendary meal that's worth mentioning. Thanks to Vinita and Nanda's brilliant idea, the group once dined with our Yoga trainer, Harinder along with me, yet another fitness buddy. It wasn't just a meal; it was a celebration of the bonds formed, the laughs shared, and the fitness journey that brought them all together. Imagine a group of sweaty warriors sitting around a table, sharing stories, and savouring food that was just as nourishing for the soul as it was for the body.

As the fitness community continues to grow and evolve, the bonds that emerge are more than just friendships—they're a testament to the power of shared experiences and the joy of making every workout a little less serious and a lot more fun. The cucumbers, the songs, the long rides, and the Yoga counts are all part of a bigger picture, one where camaraderie reigns supreme and every member contributes their unique flavour to the mix.

So, the next time I step into the Fitness Centre, I remember that I'm not just entering a gym; I'm joining a vibrant, quirky family. Each workout is a new chapter in the ongoing saga of sweat, smiles, and camaraderie. And who knows? Maybe the next surprise will involve kale chips, interpretive dance-offs, or a new nickname that's just as amusing as '*Krishna*.'

In an era dominated by digital interactions, our Fitness Centre offers a refreshing dose of face-to-face social connections. The gym becomes a hub of real-life conversations, shared jokes, and spontaneous high-fives. It's where friendships blossom amidst the clang of weights and the rhythm of cardio machines. Every workout is an opportunity to connect with others on a personal level, making the fitness journey as much about the people I meet as the goals I achieve. The gym transforms into a vibrant social scene where I am not just another member but part of a dynamic community which is constantly thinking of ways to keep the community thriving.

The Shivagange Trek - Part 1: From Dawn to Summit in Hilarious Harmony!

I was unanimously chosen to lead our first big adventure—a trek—which started with me casually tossing the idea into our group chat like a hot potato:

"Hey, who's up for a trek to Shivagange?"

Little did I know, that this spontaneous suggestion would spark so much excitement and set the wheels in motion, for an unforgettable journey!

It was meant to be a low-key suggestion, but it quickly morphed into a full-scale expedition. Five brave souls immediately jumped on board, armed with nothing but excitement and maybe a few questionable workout outfits. But as the buzz grew, so did the group. Before I knew it, our little trek had snowballed into a squad of 16 eager adventurers. It was like watching a snowball roll downhill—gathering more people, gear, and enthusiasm along the way, with just a sprinkle of madness to keep things interesting.

The date December 3, 2023, was circled, highlighted, and quite possibly adorned with glitter on all our calendars. Shivagange—the mighty mountain that seemed to call us out, daring us to conquer it! The air was thick with anticipation, almost as if we could bottle it like a morning protein shake. Excitement buzzed through us like a squirrel on too much caffeine. The scent of pre-trek jitters mingled with the unmistakable whiff of damp gym socks as we prepped to swap our usual workouts for the thrill of this epic adventure. We weren't just a fitness group; we were a fitness army ready for battle, armed with trekking poles and decked out in our brightly coloured workout gear.

The excitement was contagious. Our group chat was blowing up with messages, and the anticipation reached the kind of fever pitch usually reserved for Christmas Eve or the launch of a new superhero movie. But, of course, no adventure would be complete without a plot twist. One of our crew had to drop out last minute due to an emergency, like the universe had decided to keep us on our toes. We were down to 15 trekkers, but our spirits didn't falter. Who needs a full squad when you've got 15 eager adventurers fired up and ready to tackle Shivagange?

When the trek to Shivagange got the official green light, I knew I had to step up and handle the logistics—starting with transportation. Carpooling or renting a mini-bus? Let's be real, getting a bunch of fitness enthusiasts to a mountain at the crack of dawn requires more than a loose plan. It demands precision, foresight, and a backup plan. So, to make sure everything ran like clockwork, I did what any seasoned organiser would do: I whipped up a second WhatsApp group.

But this wasn't just any group chat. Oh no, this was a tactical strike force for transportation. After a quick internal poll, four brave souls stepped up and were anointed as our carpool captains—or carpool saviours, if you will. These chosen few were handed the sacred responsibility of ensuring our seamless journey to glory, aka the trek of a lifetime. Their mission? To organise cars, sort out fuel, and guarantee no one got left behind—unless, of course, they were late. In that case, tough luck!

Once the captains were in place, our WhatsApp group transformed into a war room. It was like watching a military operation unfold, but with fewer cameo uniforms and more emojis. Updates flowed like a river after a heavy rainstorm—constant, detailed, and at times, overwhelming. It was as if the universe had decided to turn our chat into the ultimate manual for a successful adventure. Itineraries were shared, with times so precise you could set your watch by them. Dos and don'ts were issued with the kind of authority that made you question whether you'd remembered to pack your toothbrush. And then, there were the constant reminders—so many reminders—that literally anyone would start dreaming about them. *"Remember your water bottle," "Don't forget your trekking shoes," "Bring snacks, but not too many snacks!"* It was a relentless stream of information, all aimed at ensuring we arrived at Shivagange in one piece, both physically and mentally. And through it all, one voice echoed in our ears: Mama's wisdom. *"Meticulous detailing is the key,"* and we all nodded in agreement, even if we weren't entirely sure who Mama was. It didn't matter. If Mama said it, it had to be true. And who were we to argue with Mama?

With the captains firmly in place and carpool logistics tighter than a drum, I thought of yet another idea. Because what's an epic trek without a little friendly competition? And so, in a stroke of brilliance that could only come from someone with a deep understanding of group dynamics (and a love for snazzy names), I divided our merry band of adventurers into four teams. But these weren't just any teams. Oh no, each team was given a name that would strike fear into the hearts of lesser adventurers and make us feel like we were part of something much bigger than ourselves. And thus, *Sigma Rules, Gamma Galaxy, Beta Bytes, and Alpha Alchemists* were born! These names weren't just for show; they were a reflection of our squad goals—fuel, funds, and friendship, all shared and balanced with the precision of a Swiss banker. Each team had its marching orders, and let me tell you, these teams took their names seriously.

Sigma Rules: The Enforcers of Etiquette

The Sigma Rules were like the self-appointed guardians of trek etiquette, always there to make sure we were trekking with some class. If there was a rule to follow, I bet till our last protein shake they'd be on it, making sure we all stayed in line. Their code was simple: *"If we're going to trek, we do it right."* Whether it was reminding us to keep the trail clean or making sure we stayed hydrated, they were always on point. And trust me, they had no problem giving a subtle (or not-so-subtle) nudge if someone forgot to pick up after themselves or started whining too much. Complaining wasn't part of the agenda, after all.

Gamma Galaxy: The Dreamers and Star Gazers

Then there was Gamma Galaxy. If there was ever a team that was ready to reach for the stars—literally—it was them. Gamma Galaxy was all about dreaming big and aiming high. They were the ones most likely to suggest a detour to watch the sunrise or point out constellations along the way. Their motto? *"The sky's the limit."* They were the dreamers, the ones who would pause mid-trek to take in the view and remind us all, that the journey was just as important as the destination. And if they could have trekked all the way to the stars, I can bet they would have.

Beta Bytes: The Tech Wizards

Beta Bytes, on the other hand, were the tech wizards of the group. If there was an app for trekking, they had it. If there was a gadget that could make the trek easier, they were already testing it out. Their A-game was all about bringing the latest technology to the trail. *GPS? Check. Fitness trackers? Check. A playlist that was scientifically designed to keep us motivated? Double check.* Beta Bytes were serious about their tech, and if we needed any kind of digital assistance, they were our go-to team. They may have been a little nerdy, but when we're lost in the middle of nowhere, it's the nerds who save the day.

Alpha Alchemists: The Master Planners

And finally, we had the Alpha Alchemists. These were the master planners, the ones who had a plan for everything and even a backup plan for when that plan inevitably went wrong. If Sigma Rules were the enforcers and Beta Bytes were the techies, Alpha Alchemists were the *strategists.* They were the ones who had already mapped out the entire trek, complete with pit stops and scenic overlooks. They were the ones who knew exactly how many granola bars to bring and had an extra bottle of water, just in case. Alpha Alchemists were the glue that held the whole operation together, ensuring that everything ran smoothly from start to finish.

In every well-planned adventure, there's always that one gnawing fear lurking like a storm cloud over even the most perfect itinerary: What if, on the day of the big event, the captains decided to play hide-and-seek? It's the kind of anxiety that could unravel even the most meticulously thought-out plans. But I wasn't about to let such trivialities derail our epic trek to Shivagange. I came up with a simple, fool-proof rule: the 4/4 rule, a masterclass in punctuality disguised as a guideline.

The concept was straightforward, yet bold in its simplicity: four captains, four a.m., December 3, 2023. If the captains weren't at the assembly point by 4:00 a.m. sharp, we were as good as doomed. The stakes were high, and the clock was ticking, because the rest of the team wasn't going to wait around for anyone who couldn't keep time.

Imagine this—one rogue captain rolls in late, and instead of embarking on the adventure of a lifetime, we'd be stuck belting out sad ballads on the road to Shivagange, our dreams crushed by someone's love for the snooze button. But with the 4/4 rule in place, our confidence soared. This wasn't just a rule—it was a sacred law of punctuality.

We all knew that if our captains could pull it together at the crack of dawn, the rest of us would follow suit. After all, who wanted to be the one responsible for turning our trek into a cautionary tale of what happens when you can't pry yourself out of bed on time? As the countdown to D-Day began, the 4/4 rule quickly became our mantra. It wasn't just about showing up on time; it was about setting a gold standard for excellence in time management.

Soon, it became a way of life. Dinner plans? 4/4 rule. Coffee meet-ups? 4/4 rule. Grocery shopping? Well, maybe not grocery shopping, but you get the point. The genius of this rule left us wondering why we hadn't lived by it all along.

December 3rd dawned with the kind of anticipation usually reserved for the launch of a new iPhone or the season finale of a hit TV show. The clock was ticking, and there was a sense of urgency in the air that was almost palpable. Alarms were set, reminders were pinned, and phones were charged to full capacity, because the last thing I wanted was to be that person who overslept and missed the trek of a lifetime. And then, as the minutes ticked closer to the fateful hour, the excitement reached a fever pitch. Would the captains show up on time? Would the 4/4 rule hold up under the pressure?

But of course, no epic journey would be complete without a little drama. And as fate would have it, the universe wasn't about to let us sail through this trek without a few curveballs. Just as we were all starting to feel a bit too confident, the weather decided to make a surprise appearance. Cue the gentle drizzle that began to fall at 3:00 a.m. It wasn't a downpour —just enough rain to make everyone second-guess the wisdom of setting off on a trek before dawn. The kind of drizzle that whispers, *"Are you sure about this?"* It was the universe's way of testing our resolve, to see if we were really committed to this adventure, or if we would crumble at the first sign of adversity.

But I wasn't about to let it stop us. While the rest of the crew might have been tempted to hit snooze and call it a day, my Plan B mindset kicked in faster than I could say *"weather app."* The group chat buzzed with anxious messages, and I quickly reassured everyone that a bit of drizzle wouldn't dampen our spirits. *"It's just a passing cloud,"* I declared with the confidence of someone who has had a few words with the weather gods. *"Let's hang tight and see what happens."* And so we did. As the minutes ticked by, the drizzle persisted—a gentle reminder that Mother Nature has her quirks. Just when everyone was silently praying for a break, I dropped the ultimate bombshell in the group chat at exactly 4:00 a.m.: *"I'm at the assembly point!"* It was like a triumphant battle cry declaring, *"Crisis averted! The trek is still on!"* Spirits lifted, and the WhatsApp group exploded with relieved messages. Umbrellas were abandoned, rain jackets zipped up, and with renewed enthusiasm, we geared up for the adventure of a lifetime. The drizzle, once a looming threat, had become nothing more than a minor blip in our story—a small inconvenience in the face of our unshakable resolve.

As dawn broke over the horizon, painting the sky in hues of pink and gold, our little band of adventurers began to gather at the assembly point. There was an unmistakable buzz in the air, the kind that can only come from a mix of excitement, anticipation, and a healthy dose of competitive spirit. The stage was set, and the players—each with a quirky team name that would make even the Avengers jealous—were ready to take on the day.

First up was Sigma Rules, a team that had already laid down the law when it came to trek etiquette. If there was a rulebook for how to handle a trek, these guys probably wrote it. Then there was Gamma Galaxy, a team that seemed determined to reach for the stars—literally, if they could. Leading the charge for Gamma Galaxy was none other than *Krishna* (our Mahesh), the caring soul who quickly became the hero of the hour by picking up his entire team from their respective homes. It wasn't just a lift; it was a lift in spirits, and *Krishna* earned himself enough brownie points to open a bakery. Beta Bytes came next, and while their name might suggest a group of tech-savvy trekkers who could hack their way up the mountain, they were all heart, bringing a mix of humour and resourcefulness that made them a force to be reckoned with. And then there were the Alpha Alchemists, a team with a name that promised magical transformations—likely turning their post-trek exhaustion into triumph with a few well-timed selfies and a lot of group support.

The camaraderie blossomed as everyone snapped a cool morning picture, capturing the moment before the real adventure began. It was one of those rare instances where everyone actually managed to look awake and excited in a pre-dawn photo. Captains were paired up with their respective squads, each team brimming with enthusiasm and ready for the journey ahead. Laughter echoed through the air as the teams piled into their respective vehicles, transforming the simple act of carpooling into a joyride full of jokes, jests, and just a tiny bit of nervous energy. As I set off on our journey towards Shivagange, it was clear that this wasn't just a trek—it was the start of something legendary.

As I wound my way through a maze of sleepy villages and twisty roads that seemed to lead to nowhere in particular, the question on my mind wasn't about the trek or even the weather. Nope, it was much more primal than that: *"Where the heck are I going to find breakfast out here for everyone?"*

The convoy of cars, filled with eager but increasingly hungry adventurers, resembled a pack of wolves on the hunt for their first meal of the day. As the Sun began to rise, casting a soft golden glow over the landscape, our chances of stumbling upon an open eatery seemed as slim as a dosa. The villages we passed were still fast asleep, their doors shut tight against the early morning chill, and not a single waft of food was in the air.

Just when I was beginning to consider the possibility of gnawing on my own steering wheels, there it was—a beacon of hope in the form of an open shop, bravely standing as the lone soldier of sustenance in this pre-dawn desert. I pulled in, asking others to do so and in no time, our cars lined up like a fleet of rescue vehicles that had just spotted a stranded ship. The shopkeeper, who was either a morning person or just too surprised by the sudden influx of hungry souls to protest, welcomed us with a smile that suggested he was about to have the best morning sales of his life. And then, it happened—the glorious, life-affirming smell of freshly brewed coffee and hot dosa wafted through the air like a gift from the gods. If there was ever a moment when angels sang, this was it.

Breakfast wasn't just a meal—it was a ritual, a sacred tradition that demanded reverence. Plates began to pile high with South Indian delicacies, each one more mouth-watering than the last. Crisp, golden dosas were served with a side of steaming sambar, and fluffy idlis jostled for space next to spicy chutneys. It was a feast fit for a king, or in this case, a bunch of would-be mountaineers who were definitely more concerned with fuelling up than with the upcoming climb. As I, along with others gathered around tables that seemed to materialise out of nowhere, the energy shifted. Gone were the sleepy eyes and the grumpy faces; in their place were smiles, laughter, and the kind of camaraderie that only a shared meal can bring. There was a certain magic in the air, and it wasn't just the caffeine kicking in. Maybe it was the anticipation of the trek, or maybe it was the simple joy of good food shared with good people. Whatever it was, it brought us closer together, turning a group of individuals into a team. Conversations flowed as freely as the coffee, with topics ranging from the best strategy for tackling the trek to who could eat the most dosas without regretting it later. *Spoiler alert: It turns out there's always one person who thinks they can, and they usually can't.*

Now, any seasoned trekker will tell us, that it's not just the big breakfast that matters, but the snacks I carry with me. And our group was nothing if not strategic in this department. As plates were cleared and bellies were patted in satisfaction, the real planning began—packing the Plan B snacks. Fruits and nuts, those trusty allies of the outdoorsy, were meticulously stashed away in backpacks. Bananas, apples, and oranges were carefully selected for their ability to provide instant energy, while almonds, cashews, and raisins were chosen for their snack ability and sustenance. These were the snacks that would see us through the toughest parts of the trek, the ones that would provide a much-needed boost when the mountain started to fight back. But there was a method to this madness. Packing snacks wasn't just about throwing a few things into a bag; it was an art form, a game of snack Tetris where every item had to fit just right. Too many snacks, and I'd be weighed down before I even started. Too few, and I'd be left scrounging for crumbs halfway up the mountain. But with the right balance, I could conquer anything—well, anything that didn't involve dodging monkeys trying to swipe our fruit.

With my breakfast adventure drawing to a close, I was ready. The combination of good food, great company, and meticulous snack planning had transformed me from a ragtag group of half-asleep trekkers into a well-oiled machine, ready to take on the world—or at least Shivagange. I got back into my car, spirits high and bellies full, with the unmistakable feeling that I was about to embark on something epic.

As we hit the road again, leaving behind the sleepy village and our cozy breakfast haven, a buzz of excitement filled the air. The real adventure was just beginning, and if breakfast was any indicator, the day ahead would be packed with laughter, teamwork, and maybe a bit of indigestion. But that was a problem for later. Right now, I was content—armed with snacks, fuelled by a hearty breakfast, and ready to tackle whatever lay ahead. With a start like that, how could anything possibly go wrong? Before I knew it, we reached the base of the mountain. Our first stop? A temple nestled at the foot of the climb, where we planned to seek blessings from the deity.

But this wasn't just any temple. It had that timeless, majestic feel—like it had seen more pilgrims than Google Maps had ever misled tourists. The place stood tall, serene, and ancient, almost as if it had silently judged us for the calorific indulgence we had just enjoyed at breakfast. As our convoy pulled into the temple grounds, the atmosphere shifted. The once lively chatter faded, and the bursts of laughter were replaced by a hushed reverence. For a moment, it felt like I was stepping into another era—one where mountains kept their secrets and temples offered answers. Answers we were just about to seek... right after we nailed the perfect Instagram shot, of course.

"Wait, I wasn't ready!" someone from our squad shouted, just as the unofficial photo marathon kicked off. It was like a starting gun had gone off, signalling the beginning of a chaotic yet hilarious photoshoot. Out came the smartphones, DSLRs, GoPros, and even a couple of vintage Polaroids (because, of course, someone had to be that hipster). The temple, with all its peaceful charm and ancient aura, was suddenly transformed into the backdrop for a spontaneous, full-scale photoshoot.

There were group shots, where everyone tried to cram in without stepping on each other's toes, and solo poses that ranged from the standard 'smile and wave' to the overly dramatic 'gaze into the distance like you're contemplating the meaning of life' shot. Candid moments were captured—though it's hard to call it candid when you're holding a pose for what feels like an eternity. And naturally, the classic 'holding up the temple' shot made its appearance—a masterpiece of forced perspective. When done right, it looked like we had Herculean strength, but when botched, it seemed like we were just giving directions to imaginary traffic.

The air buzzed with filters, frames, angles, and awkward stances. Someone even suggested a synchronised jump shot. What we ended up with, was a series of blurry images that resembled more of a group exorcism than a celebratory leap. But that's the magic of these moments—nothing ever goes exactly as planned, and that's precisely what makes them so unforgettable.

Despite the madness of the makeshift photo session, there was an underlying sense of calm that couldn't be ignored. Between the flashes and the filters, there were quiet moments where I could all feel the significance of the place. The temple, with its ancient walls and tranquil aura, seemed to whisper stories of those who had come before us—pilgrims, trekkers, and travellers who had stood in the very spot where we now stood, ready to take on the challenge of the mountain. There was something humbling about the experience, something that made me take a step back and really soak in the moment. It wasn't just about capturing the perfect shot; it was about capturing the essence of the journey I was about to embark on. The temple wasn't just a pit stop—it was a place to gather my thoughts, to find my centre, and to remind myself that this trek was about more than just reaching the top. It's about the journey, the camaraderie, and the memories I would make along the way.

With one final glance at the temple—a place that had given me both peace and the perfect backdrop—I turned my attention to the trail ahead. The adventure was about to begin, and with my quirky teams and its members, my newfound sense of unity, and a few hundred photos in tow, I set off on what was sure to be a day filled with challenges, triumphs, and maybe just a little bit more chaos. After all, what's an adventure without a few surprises along the way?

The Shivagange Trek – Part 2: Monkey Business, Treacherous Trails, and Whimsical Wishes

Nestled just 60 kilometres from Bangalore, Shivagange is more than just a hill—it's a multitasking marvel that wears many hats, or should we say, many faces. Standing tall at 1,368 meters above sea level, this peak is not only a trekking paradise but also a hotspot for divine interventions. Known as 'Dakshina Kashi', Shivagange is a spiritual theme park, with shrines dedicated to Shiva, Parvathi, and Ganga. There's the Gangadhareshwara Temple, the Honnadevi Temple, and a handful of spring water spots that are said to be connected to the sacred Ganges. Talk about multitasking!

The hill itself is a bit of a show-off, resembling different divine symbols depending on your viewpoint: Shiva Linga from the West, a bull from the East, a cobra from the North, and Ganesha from the South. It's like the mountain equivalent of a Rorschach Test—spiritual edition.

And if that seemed to be impressive, need to wait until Sankranti rolls around. The place transforms into a carnival of festivities, buzzing with energy, and it's probably best to steer clear of any daring treks during this time, unless you fancy sharing the trail with a few thousand extra pilgrims.

The adventure kicked off with a warning from a local Samaritan who was as sweet as sugar. With a smile as wide as the Shivagange itself, he cautioned me about the local monkey mafia that ruled the trail. Apparently, these furry bandits had a reputation for swiping anything remotely edible—or shiny. He kindly handed me a stick, which instantly transformed me from a carefree trekker into an official simian slayer (or so I thought). Armed with my new 'weapon' and feeling like the hero in a low-budget jungle movie, I was ready to face whatever cheeky primates dared to cross our path. And so, our epic journey began, with me clutching the stick like a sword in a medieval battle.

Before I got too far, I decided to loosen up with a quick warm-up routine. But this wasn't my ordinary stretch-and-go; it was more like a quirky dance party.

Picture this: 50 steps that looked like a cross between an impromptu Zumba class and a conga line gone rogue. I flailed my arms, kicked my legs, and probably confused every other trekker within a 50-meter radius. But hey, I was pumped and ready to conquer Shivagange—or at least take some epic selfies before the real climbing started. As I made my way up the trail, the temperature decided to play a game of *"Let's see who's really prepared."* The higher I climbed, the chillier it got, and that's when the true heroes in my group emerged: the backpack jugglers. Leading the charge were Roshan, Mahesh (our affectionate *Krishna*), and Avijit, each of them resembling a walking, talking, human pack mule. They weren't just carrying their own stuff—oh no, these guys were lugging around three backpacks each! I watched in awe (and slight guilt) as they trudged along, burdened like 'sherpas' on a Himalayan expedition. I threw them nods of appreciation, but deep down, I knew they deserved medals—or at least a standing ovation—for their superhuman strength and stamina.

A little further along, the trail decided to throw me a bone. I hit another pit-stop, and this time it was a section of rock-cut steps that made the ascent a bit easier. These steps, carved right into the mountain, felt like they were there to give me a breather and a sense of accomplishment. I paused to take in the view, which was nothing short of magical. The landscape stretched out before us like a scene from a postcard, all serene and misty, making the climb seem like a spiritual journey (with a lot of huffing and puffing, of course).

It was during this Zen-like moment that Aashna, our resident snack enthusiast, brought us back to reality with a very important reminder: snacks. She casually mentioned that Malini had sent along some treats, which instantly sparked joy in the group. We rummaged through our bags and found the goodies—a mix of fruits, nuts, and other healthy-ish bites. As I munched away, I realised that these snacks were more than just food; they were symbols of Malini's thoughtfulness and her unwavering belief in the power of a well-timed munchie.

In a fit of gratitude and slightly delirious humour, I decided to honour Malini in the most hilarious way possible. As a member from the squad snapped a group photo, I held her image on a stick as a prop, holding it up like a holy relic. The result? A hilarious tribute to our snack saviour that I knew would become a cherished memory, complete with the caption: *"Thanks, Malini! Powered by snacks and laughter."*

With my belly again full of snacks and my spirits lifted by our impromptu photo session, I was ready to tackle whatever Shivagange had in store for me next. The path ahead was steep, and the summit still seemed far away, but with my quirky team, a stick-wielding me, and a bunch of backpack heroes by my side, I knew we could handle anything. As I continued my ascent, the challenges became more intense, but so did my determination. The camaraderie I shared, the laughter that echoed through the trees, and the occasional playful banter made the trek more than just a physical challenge—it was an unforgettable adventure. Shivagange was testing me, but I was more than ready to rise to the occasion. After all, with a stick in hand, a backpack full of snacks, and a heart full of laughter, what could possibly go wrong? As the trail wound its way upward, my journey transformed from a casual hike into a whimsical, foggy adventure straight out of a fantasy novel. The air grew cooler, and a thick fog rolled in, wrapping everything in a misty blanket. But did I let that dampen my spirits? Absolutely not! If anything, it gave me a chance to crack more jokes about disappearing into the abyss or being swallowed by the 'Misty Mountain'—cue 'Lord of the Rings' references.

I marched on, along with others, the sound of our banter and laughter echoing through the trees. Every now and then, I passed by small shops that popped up along the trail like tiny oases, offering warm tea, snacks, and the occasional bottle of water. Hats off to these unsung heroes, the shopkeepers who somehow made it up the mountain before we did, setting up their little refreshment stands like it was no big deal. These folks were the real MVPs, serving up essentials with a side of smiles.

But not all the creatures we encountered were so hospitable. Enter the monkeys—the uninvited guests who had clearly made this trail their own. These sneaky simians had a knack for appearing out of nowhere, eyes gleaming with mischief as they scoped out any opportunity to snag a snack. I quickly realised that the monkeys were less of a nuisance and more of a monkey minefield, one wrong move and my precious banana was history. Armed with my wits (and the occasional stick), I navigated this primate gauntlet, doing my best to not provoke the little rascals while secretly hoping they didn't view me as walking vending machines.

As I ascended the ancient trail, my journey brought me to a place of profound sanctity—Olakal Theertha Temple. Nestled halfway up the mountain, this mystical cave temple is not just a place of worship but a divine sanctuary, carefully etched into the very heart of the mountain by forces beyond human comprehension. The entrance stood before us, humble yet powerful, inviting all who approached to enter with reverence and humility, as though crossing into a realm where the divine presence was palpable. It was a moment to reflect, to connect with the divine, and to seek blessings for the journey ahead.

Riddhi, ever the mindful and spiritually attuned trekker, felt a deep connection to this sacred space. She made a silent vow to revisit the temple on our return journey, recognising the significance of this sacred temple. For Riddhi, as for all of us, this was more than just a stop on the trek—it was a profound spiritual encounter that would stay with us long after we had left the mountain.

We continued our climb, eager to see what other wonders awaited us on this epic journey. It didn't take long before I was greeted by one of the trek's most breath-taking sights: a colossal statue of Shiva and Parvati, perched majestically as if they were the divine overseers of the entire landscape. Their serene expressions and the sheer scale of the statues left me in awe, a moment of quiet reverence that, of course, quickly gave way to an entirely different kind of worship—the worship of the perfect photo-op.

The cameras were out faster than you could say *"Cheese!"* and what ensued was a delightful mix of reverence and ridiculousness. Some of us, clearly feeling the spiritual vibes from our temple visit, opted for the classic meditation pose. Legs crossed, eyes closed, some tried their best to look like they had achieved inner peace, though the occasional snicker suggested otherwise.

Debolina, our resident yoga guru, was in her element. She effortlessly flowed through a series of asanas that had me wondering if I should have taken my morning stretches a bit more seriously. Watching her bend and twist with such grace, I couldn't help but give it a go. The results were... well, let's just say I won't be quitting my day jobs anytime soon. But hey, it's the effort that counts, right?

And then came the pièce de résistance: the mind-bending optical illusion yoga pose. The idea was simple—align our bodies in such a way that it looked like one person was levitating off another's head. The execution? Not so much. After several attempts, lots of wobbly legs, and more than a few giggles, we finally managed to pull it off. The photo was nothing short of epic, the kind of shot that would have our friends back home scratching their heads in disbelief and asking, *"How on Earth did you do that?"* But it wasn't just about the poses.

The scenery around me was equally worthy of capturing. With the statues standing tall against the backdrop of the misty mountains and the lush greenery, every angle offered a new perspective. Group shots, solo shots, candid shots—our cameras were working overtime. There was a kind of joyful chaos to it all, a sense that this was not just about documenting the trek, but about celebrating the sheer fun of it.

Of course, not all photo sessions went off without a hitch. There were a few near-misses—a couple of us almost took an unexpected tumble while trying to get the perfect shot. And let's not forget the wind, which decided to make a guest appearance just as I was trying to capture those serene meditation poses. It turns out, maintaining inner peace is a lot harder when I am fighting to keep my hair out of my face. Despite the occasional hiccup, the photo frenzy was a roaring success. Each click of the shutter was a moment frozen in time, a memory we would carry with us long after we had descended the mountain. The laughter, the playful teasing, the sheer joy of being together in this stunning place—it all came through in the photos. I wasn't just capturing the sights; I was capturing the spirit of the trek, the camaraderie, and the shared adventure.

As I packed up my camera and prepared to move on, there was a sense of satisfaction in the air. I had come, I had seen, and I had definitely conquered the art of the group photo. The statues of Shiva and Parvati looked on, serene as ever, as if giving their divine approval to our antics. And with that, I set off once more, ready for whatever the trail had in store for me next. The trek was far from over, and as I continued our ascent, there was an unspoken agreement among us—whatever challenges lay ahead, we would meet them with the same spirit of fun and camaraderie that had carried us this far. After all, I had already learned one of the most important lessons of the journey: sometimes, the best way to reach new heights is with a smile, a sense of humour, and a really good camera.

As I climbed higher along with the team, the fog thickened around us like a blanket of cotton candy that had gone rogue. It felt like I was trekking straight into the heavens—or maybe just into a very dramatic cloud that had decided to put on a show for me. The landscape started playing tricks on me, with trees and rocks appearing and disappearing like characters in a spooky movie. One minute, I was walking beside a friendly-looking boulder, and the next, it vanished into the mist, leaving me wondering if it was ever there at all. Was it eerie? Absolutely. Was it exhilarating? You bet. It was the kind of atmosphere that made me feel like I was starring in an epic adventure—if that adventure involved a lot of tripping over your own feet.

Of course, the trail had no intention of making things easy for me. It wasn't just a stroll in the park; it was more like a high-stakes obstacle course designed by someone with a twisted sense of humour. The path became steeper and slicker with every step, as if it had been polished by a thousand mischievous mountain spirits. And the rocks? Oh, they had their own agenda, conspiring to twist our ankles at every opportunity. If rocks could laugh, these ones would definitely be chuckling every time I slipped.

The fog, now my constant companion, decided to add to the drama by reducing visibility to about two feet. If I could see my own hand in front of my face, I were one of the lucky ones. More often than not, someone would stumble on a loose stone or get a face full of wet leaves, which led to a lot of impromptu interpretive dance moves as I tried to keep my balance. But instead of grumbling, I embraced the chaos with the kind of enthusiasm that only comes from knowing I'll laugh about it later. *"Embrace the mud!"* someone shouted, and we all cheered, like a group of very muddy, very enthusiastic cheerleaders. The terrain was challenging, no doubt about it, but my spirits were unshakeable—mostly because I was too busy enjoying the beauty around me to be bothered by a few bumps and bruises.

And then, there were the moments of sheer, delightful confusion. The trail, ever the trickster, seemed to enjoy splitting into two or, even worse, disappearing altogether into the fog. *"Which way now?"* someone would call out, sparking a lively debate. Left or right? Up or down? Forward or backward? In the end, we'd pick a direction more by gut feeling than any actual logic, because really, what's a trek without a little detour? Or, in my case, several. Getting lost became part of the adventure, and I embraced it with open arms (and occasionally open arms that were flailing wildly as we stumbled down the wrong path). After all, detours are where the best stories are born. I'd follow the sound of laughter echoing through the fog, trusting that as long as the group is stuck together, I'd find my way—eventually. And if not, well, I'd at least have a great time trying.

The adventure that was sold to us as a "moderate" trek—a term as misleading as *"Just one more episode"*—began with the usual mixture of excitement and blissful ignorance.

"How hard can it be?" Riddhi and Rohan mused, their optimism bubbling over like a freshly popped bottle of soda. They turned towards me, my group's de facto trek guru, for some insider information.

I didn't sugarcoat it: *"From the statue of Shiva and Parvati to the hill's peak, it's more of an upward rollercoaster than a leisurely stroll."*

My warning, however, did nothing to dampen our spirits. After all, who wouldn't want to ride a rollercoaster that only goes up? The kind where my quads scream louder than I do. The trail steepened faster than a plot twist in a soap opera. One moment, I was walking on what feels like a gentle incline, and the next, I am practically scaling a wall. And those steps—calling them steps would be generous. They were more like uneven ledges, each one narrower than the last, and just wide enough for me to question all my life choices. It wasn't long before I realised that this wasn't just a trek; it was a full-blown leg day workout disguised as a spiritual journey.

But what's a trek without a challenge, right? Despite the fog so thick I could spread it on toast, my enthusiasm remained undeterred. Visibility was down to about two feet, which meant that everyone's view was limited to the back of the person in front of them and the next step they were about to trip over. If anyone could've seen our faces, they'd have seen a mix of determination and mild panic, the kind usually reserved for last-minute exam preparations. Thank the trekking gods for the railings—those cold, metal lifelines were the only things keeping us from a one-way ticket to the bottom. I clung to them with the same desperation usually reserved for Wi-Fi in a crowded cafe. Without those railings, this trek would have turned into the kind of story I hear on late-night news channels, complete with dramatic re-enactments and ominous background music.

And just when I thought we had enough on our plates—with the fog, the steps, and the relentless upward climb—the local wildlife decided to make an appearance. Enter the monkeys, the uninvited guests to our uphill party. These furry freeloaders were everywhere, hopping from railing to railing like they were auditioning for the next 'Planet of the Apes' sequel. Their keen interest in our bags was unnerving, especially when one particularly bold monkey set its sights on Rohit. Poor Rohit stood frozen as the monkey rifled through his bag like a TSA agent on a power trip. The suspense was palpable as the monkey inspected the contents with the kind of focus usually seen in bomb squads. Toffees and bubblegum? The monkey's disdain was evident as it discarded them with a sniff, clearly unimpressed by Rohit's snack selection. It was the primate equivalent of getting socks for Christmas!

Despite the monkey business (pun totally intended), I managed to keep my energy up, thanks in no small part to Avijit's impromptu exercise routines. While I was content to use the trek itself as a workout, Avijit decided to throw in some quad and hamstring stretches for good measure. If only the monkeys had joined in—they might have learned the benefits of a good stretch before their next bag inspection.

As I neared the summit, a chilly breeze hit us like a surprise ice bucket challenge, reminding me that I was indeed ascending to new heights—literally. It was jacket weather now, and the sudden drop in temperature was both refreshing and a bit alarming.

"How much higher is this peak?" someone muttered, pulling their jacket tighter. The summit was tantalisingly close, and with each step, the anticipation grew. The first thing that greeted us at the top was the colossal Nandi statue, carved from rock and standing guard like a benevolent bouncer. The air here was thick with reverence, a stark contrast to the giggly chaos of our ascent. I removed my shoes, out of respect for the sacred ground—a close-up with Nandi himself.

Here's a nugget of wisdom: If someone whispers their wish into Nandi's ears and have been a decent human being (i.e., haven't pushed anyone off the trail), legend has it that the wish will be granted. It's like a mystical drive-thru for wish fulfilment, no app necessary. We took turns whispering our secrets and desires, feeling a strange mix of hope and amusement at the ritual. After all, what harm could it do to ask for a little divine intervention? With my wishes made, I ventured behind the bull statue, where the real fun began. The railings here offered not just support, but an adrenaline rush that rivalled any amusement park ride. With no solid ground beneath me, balancing on these metal bars was like walking a tightrope over a foggy abyss. It was the ultimate test of nerve and balance, and I was all too happy to take it on—more confidently than others.

A few more cautious steps and I arrived at Shanthala Point with my team, a viewpoint named after the legendary Bharatanatyam dancer queen. The view, or what I imagined would be the view, was completely obscured by the fog, making me feel like I was standing on the edge of the world. The air was cool, crisp, and filled with that rare sense of achievement that comes from pushing myself just a little further than I thought possible. I was above the clouds—literally and figuratively.

But no summit celebration is complete without a snack break, and I was more than ready to dig into the supplies brought by my team. Deepika, Rashmi, Aashna, Kavita, Benny, Rudra, Bakshi, and the rest of the crew wasted no time pulling out noodles, chips, and various treats from their bags.

Despite the cold, there was no shortage of willpower when it came to eating. We huddled together, sharing food, stories, and the warmth of camaraderie, all while trying to strike the perfect pose for our summit selfies. The scene was a mix of shivering bodies and wide grins, as everyone attempted to capture the foggy majesty of the moment on their phones. It was the kind of experience that would soon flood social media feeds with hashtags like #AboveTheClouds, #TrekGoals, and #NandiKnowsBest. The fog may have obscured the view, but it couldn't dampen our spirits.

The Shivagange Trek – Part 3: Krishna's Concoction and the Journey Back

Just when I thought our adventure had hit its peak (both literally and figuratively), Mahesh—whom we fondly call *Krishna*—decided that the trek wasn't complete without a culinary experiment that would make even the bravest of us question our life choices.

It began innocently enough. Riddhi, ever the organised one, had prepared some rotis and bhindi. Rashmi, channelling her inner fruit vendor, had brought along some bananas. A normal person might have simply enjoyed these items as they were, but Mahesh was not a normal person. No, Mahesh was a culinary maverick, a man determined to push the boundaries of what should and should not be mixed in a bowl.

With a gleam in his eye that can only be described as mischievous—or perhaps mildly dangerous—Mahesh surveyed his ingredients like a mad scientist on the brink of a breakthrough. Bananas, bhindi, rotis, and... badam milk smoothie. A lesser man might have stopped there, content with the knowledge that some things are better left uncombined. But Mahesh, ever the innovator, saw potential in this chaotic collection of foodstuffs. Without a moment's hesitation, he mashed the bananas with the enthusiasm of someone who'd just discovered a hidden talent. Next, he poured in the Badam Milk smoothie, stirring it with the kind of gusto usually reserved for competitive eating contests. The result? A thick, beige concoction that looked like something I might find in a science lab—under a microscope.

"Voilà!" Mahesh declared, presenting his creation to the group with a flourish that would make a French chef blush. But instead of applause, Mahesh was met with the sound of feet shuffling and the sudden disappearance of his audience. Like leaves in a windstorm, we scattered, each of us suddenly remembering urgent tasks that simply couldn't wait. Benny needed to find a signal to check on the score of a cricket match that wasn't even happening. Rohit was determined to inspect the nearby bushes for, well, anything. Deepika was certain she'd dropped her contact lenses despite wearing glasses.

Mahesh, however, was unfazed. He stood there, spoon in hand, the picture of culinary pride, as he surveyed the empty space where his friends had once stood. It was as if he couldn't quite understand why no one was leaping at the chance to taste his gastronomic masterpiece. After all, wasn't food just about mixing things you like? Bananas—good. Badam Milk—great. Bhindi? Well, it's a vegetable, so healthy. Why wouldn't they taste good together?

In his defence, Mahesh had always been the adventurous type, whether it was on the trail or in the kitchen. He was the kind of person who would add an extra spoon of chilli powder to a dish just to "see what happens." But this? This was another level of culinary courage, and we weren't sure if we should admire it or report it to the authorities.

Eventually, the bravest of the bunch, Roshan, stepped forward, lured by Mahesh's earnest enthusiasm. *"Alright, Krishna,"* Roshan said, using Mahesh's nickname as a sign of camaraderie, *"Let's see what you've got."* Roshan picked up a spoon, hesitated, then took a deep breath—like a man about to dive into shark-infested waters.

With all eyes on him (from a safe distance, of course), Roshan dipped the spoon into the concoction and raised it to his lips. There was a collective holding of breath, the kind of tension usually reserved for the final moments of a reality show. Roshan tasted, chewed, and then... the reaction. His face contorted in a way that could only be described as 'trying to smile while swallowing regret.' The taste test ended with a cough, a forced thumbs-up, and a quick exit to the nearest bush. Mahesh, ever the optimist, took Roshan's reaction in stride. *"It's an acquired taste,"* he said, as if his creation was a rare delicacy misunderstood by the masses. *"You'll come around."*

But the group, now wary of Mahesh's culinary ambitions, had already made up their minds. No one else was willing to risk their taste buds on what could only be described as a smoothie-bhindi hybrid from a parallel universe. Despite the chaos, Mahesh couldn't have been more pleased. He'd succeeded in his mission to shake things up—literally—and that was all that mattered. As the day went on, Mahesh's concoction became the stuff of legends, with exaggerated tales of its potency making the rounds. Some claimed it could fuel a trekker for days, others joked it was the secret to growing chest hair. But one thing was certain: Mahesh's madcap culinary experiment had given me a story I'd be laughing about, for years to come.

After the grand gastronomic disaster that was *Krishna's* concoction, we began our descent from the summit. The return trip down was a relief; it was easier than the climb up, though still required some cautious navigation. The narrow path wound its way down the mountain, presenting a different set of challenges that we tackled with a mixture of caution and carefree banter. The laughter that echoed through the rocky trail was as refreshing as the cool mountain breeze, as we rehashed every absurd moment from our trek.

As I made my way down, I stumbled upon a delightful surprise: a series of makeshift kiosks that seemed to have sprouted from the mountainside like magic. These little stalls offered everything from icy bottles of water to fresh, crunchy cucumbers to sizzling hot pakodas! It felt like I had accidentally wandered into a mountain carnival, where the vendors were seasoned pros at tempting weary trekkers. The smell of those golden, crispy pakodas was almost enough to make us forget the trauma of *Krishna's* concoction—almost.

Riddhi, our ever-enthusiastic spiritual seeker, had an epiphany. She remembered her promise to visit the mystical 'Olakal Theertha Temple', which was nestled halfway down the mountain. Known for its magical water spring, this hidden gem was said to offer spiritual blessings to those who made the pilgrimage. With *Krishna's* culinary catastrophe still fresh in our minds, the promise of divine intervention seemed like just the thing we needed. So, with a mix of curiosity and hope for some miraculous relief, I agreed and requested the team to make the detour. Everyone eagerly agreed. Upon arriving at the temple, I quickly discovered that we weren't the only ones with the bright idea of visiting this spiritual hotspot. The queue stretched out longer than a Monday morning traffic jam, a testament to the temple's popularity. After a brief wait and a modest entrance fee, I ventured inside the cave temple, which was cool, dimly lit, and exuded an aura of ancient mystery.

The playful banter and light-heartedness that had accompanied me so far gently faded away, replaced by a profound sense of awe and respect. The cave was designed with a unique architectural quirk: it required taller visitors to bend at an almost impossible 6:45 clock angle to navigate through. While the shorter members of our group breezed through with the ease of a well-rehearsed dance move, the taller ones resembled a collection of contorted paperclips. If the temple had a height restriction, I was clearly pushing the limits.

Every step I took, felt like a step deeper into the sacred mystery of the mountain, drawing us closer to the divine. Deeper within, I arrived at a hallowed chamber. In its centre lay a small, circular opening in the rock floor, unassuming yet imbued with an indescribable spiritual energy. It was here that the legend of Olakal Theertha came to life—a legend passed down through generations, whispered by the devout and revered by all who sought the blessings of the divine.

The legend spoke of the sacred waters that flowed beneath this very spot, waters that were believed to be a manifestation of the holy river Ganga. It was said that only those who were pure of heart, free from the stains of sin and filled with the light of goodness, could reach into the opening and touch these crystalline waters. To make contact with the sacred waters was not merely a physical act; it was a spiritual experience, one that would cleanse the soul and bring peace to the seeker. This purification was seen as a divine gift, a testament to the grace and mercy of the gods. As I stood in the presence of this sanctified chamber, I was moved by the weight of the moment. The stillness of the temple, the soft murmurs of prayer, and the subtle fragrance of incense created an atmosphere of deep contemplation and reverence.

After our spiritually invigorating detour, we resumed our journey toward the base along with others, where the growling of our stomachs had reached a crescendo. It was 12:30 p.m., and the pressing issue of the moment wasn't enlightenment but lunch. Our conversations quickly shifted from divine revelations to more earthly concerns, and before I knew it, we had a full-blown debate on our hands. Picture a group of starving trekkers turned into culinary critics, each passionately pitching their favourite lunch spots as if they were auditioning for a role on a top food reality show.

Suddenly, everyone had an opinion, and the suggestions started flying faster than we had descended from the hilltop. The debate took on the intensity of a high stakes cooking competition, with each contestant determined to outdo the others in gastronomic expertise. The variety of options was dizzying—there were calls for everything from local dhabas to international cuisine, with a few wildcards thrown in for good measure.

Amid the flurry of suggestions, Mowli, our ever-resourceful trek mate, emerged as the voice of reason. With the wisdom of someone who had clearly put a lot of thought into post-trek dining, Mowli suggested 'DeMandarin', a restaurant known for its broad menu that could cater to everyone's tastes, from die-hard vegetarians to the most carnivorous of carnivores. It was as if Mowli had just proposed the culinary equivalent of world peace. After a moment of collective reflection—and the undeniable allure of DeMandarin's mouth-watering menu—the group agreed. The decision was met with unanimous approval, a rare moment of unity in the otherwise chaotic world of post-trek lunch plans. The mere thought of food seemed to inject us with a new burst of energy. My pace quickened like others, and suddenly, the aches and pains of the morning's trek faded into the background. I descended with a renewed sense of purpose, my legs seemingly powered by the promise of a hearty meal. It was as if the idea of lunch had miraculously turned me into a well-oiled marching band member, each step perfectly in sync with the rumbling of my belly.

Upon reaching the base, the leaders of my eclectic trekking groups—Sigma Rules, Gamma Galaxy, Beta Bytes, and Alpha Alchemists—quickly rallied their troops for the final leg of our adventure: the march to DeMandarin. It was like herding cats, only these cats were particularly hungry and had just survived a mountain climb. The captains were in full command mode, each determined to get their teams to the restaurant as quickly as possible before the hunger turned into a mutiny.

However, not everyone was focused solely on food. Self, being the captain of the Alpha Alchemists, had a different kind of sustenance in mind. My team, known for their love of a good time and a well-timed detour, had spotted a nearby liquor shop. For me and my crew, the call of the bottle was too strong to resist.

It was like watching a moth drawn to a flame—except in this case, the flame was a neon sign promising cold beer and strong spirits. With a wink and a nod, I signalled to my team that a quick pit stop was in order. As the rest of the team headed toward DeMandarin, I led my merry band of Alchemists on a little side quest of our own. The rest of the group was blissfully unaware of our detour, still high on the prospect of a satisfying lunch, but my team was about to embark on an entirely different kind of culinary adventure.

As others made their eager march toward DeMandarin, visions of a well-deserved feast dancing in their heads, the phones suddenly erupted with group notifications. I was on the line, my voice carrying the laid-back vibe of someone who had just stumbled upon a hidden treasure. "*Hey, guys,*" I began, as if I was merely suggesting a casual stopover, "*We took a little detour. Found a liquor shop. Wanna join?*"

Now, let's be honest—after a trek that had already included holy detours, *Krishna's* concoction that flirted with food poisoning, and some impromptu yoga poses in a cave, my proposition was nothing short of irresistible. Who could say no to a little 'liquid courage' after all that? With the drop of a pin, my path shifted, and by the time some of the team members arrived at the scene, my team Alpha Alchemists was well ahead of others, not just in spirit but 'with spirits'. We were already a few pegs deep, looking like we were about to turn this pit stop into the main event. With the flair of a seasoned bartender at a five-star resort (or maybe just a frat party), I generously handed out beer bottles to the latecomers while keeping a couple of whiskey bottles tucked away like a secret weapon. The liquor shop had become the site of an impromptu party, complete with laughter, bottle clinking, and the kind of camaraderie that only grows stronger with every sip.

My spirits—both figuratively and quite literally—were sky-high as I finally managed to steer our slightly tipsy group toward the restaurant. Once we arrived at DeMandarin, the fun didn't just carry on; it kicked into high gear. I slipped effortlessly into the role of the group's unofficial bartender, and the whiskey I'd been saving made its grand debut. What was supposed to be a simple lunch quickly turned into the next chapter of my trek's unforgettable adventure, with the restaurant becoming the stage for yet another round of mischief.

Plates of food began to arrive, but the real star of the meal was the never-ending stream of stories, each one more outrageous than the last. What unfolded next was nothing short of culinary chaos—in the best way possible. Platters piled with butter naan, bowls brimming with spicy noodles, and plates stacked with every delicacy DeMandarin could whip-up all across the table with the urgency of a Black Friday Sale! As the food kept coming, so did the stories—each one more exaggerated and hilarious than the last. Someone, possibly emboldened by the whiskey, recounted the moment Riddhi nearly knocked herself out trying to navigate the temple cave, drawing gasps and guffaws from all sides. Another brave soul dared to describe *Krishna's* infamous concoction, dubbing it 'a dish best served never,' which prompted a round of applause and more than a few relieved sighs that none of us had succumbed to food poisoning.

The restaurant buzzed with our infectious laughter, the kind that turns heads and raises eyebrows, the warmth of camaraderie enveloped us, turning every bite into a shared victory, every sip into a celebratory toast, and every joke into a treasure that I'd revisit for years to come. DeMandarin wasn't just serving the lunch; it was dishing out the kind of memories that would become the stuff of legends.

By the time I leaned back in my chair, fully sated and just a little bit wobbly, I couldn't help but reflect on the sheer absurdity of the day's events. What began as a simple trek had morphed into a grand odyssey—complete with divine detours, questionable culinary experiments, and the kind of spontaneous shenanigans that I just can't make up. As I surveyed the aftermath of our lunch, I knew one thing for sure: this was no ordinary meal; it was the grand finale to a day that none of us would soon forget. And as for what comes next? Well, I'll just have to top this legendary lunch with an even more outrageous adventure next time. Cheers to that!

As the sun began its descent, casting a warm, golden hue over DeMandarin, the time had come for my final ritual: the farewell photos. Of course, I couldn't just leave without capturing the day's glory—especially after such a memorable trek. It was 5 pm, and the golden hour had never looked better. The restaurant, with its picturesque setting, provided the perfect backdrop for our group's last hurrah.

I got our teams assembled like a bunch of eager school kids on picture day, each of us vying for the best spot in the frame. *"Everyone say 'Krishna's Concoction!'"* someone joked, which resulted in a chorus of laughter, followed by some hilariously exaggerated poses. There were the classic group huddles, the mandatory 'jump shot' (which took three tries to perfect), and even a few candid moments of everyone bursting into laughter at the ridiculousness of it all.

As the phones and cameras snapped away, what began as a casual photoshoot quickly escalated into a mini-event of its own. Each group—Sigma Rules, Gamma Galaxy, Beta Bytes, and Alpha Alchemists—struck their signature poses, showcasing their team pride. The Alpha Alchemists, still buzzing from their earlier liquid pit stop, insisted on a series of "cheers" photos, complete with imaginary glasses raised in mock celebration.

Once the photo frenzy wrapped up, it was time to pile back into our respective cars. The group captains did their head counts, ensuring no one was left behind—although there was a brief moment of panic when someone noticed *Krishna* was still inside, trying to sweet-talk the restaurant staff into revealing their secret recipes. With everyone finally accounted for, I gathered the team to begin our journey back home.

As the car rides became quieter, with the exhaustion finally setting in, there was a collective realisation of what an extraordinary day it had been. The laughter and chaos had drawn me and everyone closer together, creating bonds that could only be forged through shared experiences—particularly ones that involved questionable cooking and unexpected detours. Driving home, I found myself replaying the day's events in my mind. The sense of achievement from reaching the summit, the thrill of the descent, and the sheer joy of being surrounded by such a fantastic group of friends. It was a day filled with everything that makes life worth living: adventure, laughter, and the kind of camaraderie that makes even the most challenging moments feel like pure fun.

As I finally pulled into my driveway, a smile spread across my face. This was a trek that would go down in history—not just for the hike itself, but for the memories I created along the way. And while the physical journey had come to an end, the stories would live on, shared over many more treks, dinners, and perhaps a few more of *Krishna's* concoctions (though hopefully not anytime soon).

Bruised, Bold, and Blissful: The Fab4's Daredevil Dash Odyssey

As the Sun crept over the horizon on December 17, 2023, the Fab4—who I had dramatically rebranded as the Dare Devils 4 (DD4)—were anything but composed. With only eight hours left before we faced the notorious Daredevil Dash obstacle run in Bangalore, my emotions were a heady mix of excitement, anticipation, and that mild panic you get before a major exam or an unexpected visit from the in-laws. But the DD4 weren't your typical weekend warriors. No, we were a fearless quartet united by a thirst for adventure, a sprinkle of masochism, and a healthy dose of caffeine. Leading this chaotic crew was none other than yours truly—the self-proclaimed captain. With the same over-the-top enthusiasm that makes late-night infomercials seem convincing, I had roped my friends into this wild ride, spinning tales that made it sound like I was a seasoned Daredevil Dash veteran.

It was up to me to rally Aashna, Promila, and Rohit to the venue by 6:30 a.m. Not that they had much of a choice; I had somehow morphed into the group's overzealous early bird, not only catching the worm but also delivering an impromptu motivational speech about it. This early start wasn't driven by excitement so much as necessity, giving us enough time to navigate whatever chaos awaited us—whether it be the battle for parking, mentally preparing for the physical ordeal ahead, or squeezing in a last-minute pep talk.

The ride to the event was a tale of contrasts. I was buzzing with anticipation, already imagining the glorious mud-splattered victory photo that would soon find its way onto my social media. Meanwhile, Aashna and Promila were huddled together, strategizing like battlefield commanders preparing for an epic campaign. Their focus was intense—every obstacle already mapped out in their minds, every potential pitfall accounted for. They didn't just follow the rules; they practically invented them. Their conversation sounded like a tactical briefing: *"We'll hit the Climb Crusher first, then go for the monkey bars using a swing-swing-catch technique, and conserve energy for the final sprint."* It was clear they weren't leaving anything to chance.

In stark contrast, Rohit and I took a more relaxed approach, channelling our inner philosophers. I echoed - *"Joh hoga dekha jayega!"* philosophy—a mantra that roughly translates to, *"Eh, we'll cross that bridge when we get to it."* My approach was the kind of laid-back wisdom that made them the perfect balance to Aashna and Promila's calculated intensity.

In no time, we reached the venue, parked, and made the 500-meter walk to the event arena—a wild wonderland built for the fearless and perhaps a little crazy. The obstacles ahead were daunting, but the collective adrenaline of the crowd was even more intense. And there we were, my crew and I—proudly known as the Fab4 or Dare Devils 4—stepping into this electrifying playground with a blend of excitement, wide-eyed wonder, and just a hint of pre-race jitters.

First off, let me talk about the baggage counters—an oasis of sanity in a desert of pre-race jitters. They were like the VIP lounges of the event, where I could drop off my existential dread along with my bags. Nearby, the medical assistance canopies stood like knightly sentinels, ready to spring into action at the first sign of an epic tumble or a twisted ankle. And for those who like to mix a little retail therapy with their physical exertion, the Daredevil Dash merchandise tents were a treasure trove of all things branded. From bandanas that screamed "I love pain" to T-shirts boasting your newfound endurance superpowers, these stalls had it all. It was like the Olympics meets a rock concert, with a side of "You've earned this T-shirt!"

Ah, the warm-up dance area—an unmissable spectacle of flailing limbs and questionable dance moves. Imagine a sea of people moving in what could only be described as a mass audition for 'America's Got No Talent.' There was an undeniable energy in the air, a sort of chaotic ballet where everyone seemed to be channelling their inner caffeinated squirrel. Watching it was like witnessing a live action cartoon where the characters had swapped their usual antics for enthusiastic attempts at synchronised chaos. Strangely enough, this spectacle of sporadic flailing set the perfect tone for the day's absurdity. If anyone could make a 25-foot honeycomb structure look like a giant puzzle from a dystopian board game, it was me.

Speaking of the honeycomb, let's just say it was a sight to behold. Towering over me like a giant, sticky Rubik's cube from a twisted carnival, it stood as a foreboding teaser of the obstacles to come. It was a piece of architecture so deviously designed; it made me wonder if the creators had a sideline in ancient torture devices.

And amidst all this, there was Reema—our Yoga buddy and beacon of positivity. She was there to cheer us on, her enthusiasm a bright spot in the swirling chaos. If good luck vibes were a currency, Reema would've been a billionaire. Her cheers were like motivational glitter, adding a bit of sparkle to our buzzing anticipation. Honestly, her presence was so uplifting, we almost wanted to wrap her up and take her with us as a good-luck charm.

As the clock inched closer to 8 a.m., signalling the start of Wave-C (obstacle slot), I huddled in 'Farhan's Den'—a corner of the arena named after the charismatic founder of Daredevil Dash , Farhan Khan . Imagine a motivational speaker with the power to sell ice to an Eskimo, and you've got Farhan. His speech was nothing short of a pep talk on steroids, leaving me feeling like I could take on a herd of charging rhinos armed with nothing but sheer willpower. His words hit me like a double espresso shot straight to the soul, priming me for the upcoming obstacle course with a level of excitement usually reserved for children on Christmas morning. With Farhan's inspiring words still echoing in my ears, it was time.

I leaped into action with the kind of dramatic flourish that would make a Hollywood director proud. With a resounding *"HALA BOL!"* that could've roused the spirits of past marathon runners, us Fab4 launched into the fray. Our 5 km obstacle course, which stretched out before us like a serpentine nightmare, was our battlefield. The course, adorned with 15 devilish obstacles, was set to test our mettle and stamina in ways we hadn't imagined. It was like a roller coaster, but with more mud, more sweat, and a lot less seat belts.

With adrenaline pumping and spirits soaring, I was ready to dive into the devilish delights of the Daredevil Dash . The course was a wild buffet of obstacles—each one more daring than the last, each one promising its own special brand of challenge and mayhem. As I set off, I knew one thing for sure: this was going to be yet another unforgettable adventure, filled with laughter, triumphs, and probably a few mud-stained souvenirs.

The Fab4 were ready, equipped with an insatiable appetite for challenges and a camaraderie that turned every hurdle into a shared adventure. And as I took my first steps onto the course, I couldn't help but think that, no matter what happened, I am in for one heck of a ride!

Having barely caught my breath from the thrilling hustle of the Arena of Anticipation, the Fab4, our brave brigade of obstacle aficionados, ventured into the heart of the challenge. Just one kilometre into my quest, I was greeted by the first formidable hurdle: *The Crawl of Fame*. Imagine a net strung low over the ground, daring me to slither beneath it with the kind of determination usually reserved for covert military operations. It was as if a group of ants had been assigned a mission to crawl under a particularly convoluted picnic blanket.

"Remember," bellowed the ever-serious marshal. *"No lifting fellow runners!"*

With this sage advice ringing in my ears, I plunged into the net with the enthusiasm of kids let loose in a ball pit. Armed with nothing but sheer willpower and a questionable amount of grace, I dived under the net. Picture me: my belly scraping the Earth, arms flailing in a desperate attempt to avoid becoming a human tumbleweed. It was a blend of crawling, wriggling, and what could only be described as interpretive dance.

Aashna, our intrepid leader, emerged with a determined scowl that could have melted steel. Promila, with her air of cheeky triumph, seemed to revel in the muddy challenge. Rohit sported a look of bemused disbelief, as if he'd just woken up from a nap and discovered he was in the middle of a live-action cartoon. And then there was me, who made my exit with a flourish worthy of a pro wrestler sliding out of the ring. My dramatic exit was not just a departure from the *Crawl of Fame,* but a full-blown performance.

With the *Crawl of Fame* behind me, I regrouped with my team, my spirits high and my body smeared with a fashion statement known as "muddy chic."

The next obstacle on the adventure was the *Climb Crusher*—an imposing vertical challenge that dared me to scale its height. It was like the universe had decided to throw in a literal wall just to see if I were really as motivated as I claimed to be.

I approached the wall with the confidence of seasoned climbers and the bravado of people who'd just successfully navigated a maze of mud. Thanks to Avijit's shoulder exercises at our Fitness Centre, which were touted as the key to wall-scaling prowess, I tackled the 6-foot barrier with the grace of mountain goats on an espresso high. Avijit's regimen had clearly worked wonders, as I powered up the wall with an agility that was nothing short of impressive. One by one, we ascended the wall, each of us taking turns to display our climbing skills. I reached the top and promptly seized my first Red Bull. My energy burst was so potent it could have powered a small city. The Fab4 was soon buzzing with a frenetic enthusiasm that made the *Climb Crusher* feel like a mere warm-up compared to what lay ahead.

Next on the obstacle agenda was the aptly named *Sky Stalker*—a pole-climbing spectacle that had me feeling like I was about to audition for the circus. The goal? Climb 15 feet above the ground on a pole that seemed to stretch all the way to the Stratosphere! It was the kind of challenge that made me question my life choices, but then Promila, with her signature cheeky grin, piped up, *"Piece of cake! It's just a walk in the clouds!"* Naturally, I nodded in wild agreement, though inwardly, I was already picturing myself dangling from that pole like human wind chimes. But if Promila could tackle it with such nonchalance, I had to at least pretend I was equally fearless. After all, how hard could it be to climb a pole in front of your closest friends who were fully prepared to either cheer you on or laugh hysterically at your inevitable struggles?

We took turns to climb the *Sky Stalker*. Promila, of course, was the first to ascend, scaling the pole with the ease of a seasoned monkey. *"See? Nothing to it!"* she called down, her voice laced with playful bravado. I followed along with the rest, each with our own style—some more graceful than others. There were a few wobbles, a couple of near-slips, and more than one moment of hanging on for dear life, but I made it to the top, my pride mostly intact.

But just when I thought I had conquered the skies, the next challenge loomed before me like something straight out of an action movie. Enter *Peak Freak* , a colossal 50-foot structure that combined net climbing, truss crossing, and a serious need for bravery. If *Sky Stalker* had me feeling like circus performers, *Peak Freak* was about to turn me into full-fledged stunt doubles. The climb up the net was a test of endurance and nerves. Each step brought me higher, and the ground seemed to disappear beneath me. The wind picked up, adding to the drama, and I clung to the net like determined spiders, focused on not looking down. The truss crossing was another beast entirely—like walking a tightrope, except the rope was a metal beam, and the fall below was something I preferred not to think about.

After what felt like an eternity, I finally made it to the top, my muscles screaming in protest but my spirits soaring with triumph. The view from up there was nothing short of breathtaking—if I could catch my breath, that is. I was on top of the world, quite literally, and it called for a photo op. But Aashna and Rohit, never ones to pass up an opportunity for mischief, had other plans. Just as I was about to snap the perfect shot, the mischievous duo pulled off a photo-bombing masterpiece. Aashna threw up bunny ears while Rohit executed a perfectly timed jump that sent him flying into the frame like a human comet. The result? A chaotic, hilarious, and utterly unforgettable group photo that perfectly captured the spirit of the day.

As I descended from the *Peak Freak* , still buzzing from the adrenaline and the laughter, I couldn't help but feel a sense of camaraderie that only comes from facing fears together—and maybe a bit of shared insanity too. Because when I was 50 feet up in the air with nothing but a net and a prayer, there's no room for anything but trust, humour, and the willingness to embrace every crazy, wonderful moment.

With Promila finally catching up to our motley crew, the Fab4 was ready to face the next challenge—*Tumble Thunder* . When I first laid eyes on *Tumble Thunder* , I knew I was about to face an obstacle that could only be described as a circus act designed by someone who really, really hated the concept of equilibrium. Imagine, if you will, a horseshoe-shaped contraption that looked like it had been plucked straight out of a roller coaster blueprint—minus the safety features. It wobbled, it swayed, and it promised a show of acrobatics that would make even circus clowns pause in admiration. Or perhaps horror. The setup was less 'balance beam' and more 'tightrope walk over a pit of chaos.' With a structure like that, the only certainty was that there would be tumbles, stumbles, and perhaps a few moments of grace under pressure—or lack thereof.

As I mustered my courage to tackle the beast of an obstacle, the atmosphere was buzzing with anticipation. I was eagerly awaiting the arrival of Promila, our newest recruit, who was about to join me in this test of balance and bravery. And because no great challenge is complete without a social media shout-out, I took a moment to snap a few photos. After all, what's an obstacle run without an Instagram post showcasing my best "I'm about to topple" faces?

Promila, looking like a cross between a determined adventurer and someone who might be considering a career in extreme sports, approached the *Tumble Thunder* with a mix of steely resolve and palpable trepidation. It was clear she was as ready as she'd ever be to face this wobbling monstrosity. With a deep breath and a series of shouts and cheers from the sidelines—ranging from motivational mantras to comedic quips—she took her first step onto the obstacle. I watched with bated breath as Promila wobbled, swayed, and then somehow managed to keep herself upright. From my vantage point, it was a masterclass in tension and comic relief. I couldn't resist adding my own running commentary, which had all the hallmarks of a stand-up routine mixed with a cheerleading squad's enthusiasm.

As Promila made it to the other side of the *Tumble Thunder* , the rest of the crew members erupted into applause. It was less about her remarkable feat of staying upright and more about our collective achievement of holding in our laughter long enough to give her a round of applause! We cheered with all the gusto of a crowd at a comedy show, celebrating not just Promila's successful crossing but our ability to keep it together as we watched her navigate the obstacle with a blend of grace and occasional flailing.

The celebration continued as I marvelled at the fact that none of us had ended up as a muddy heap in the water below. The *Tumble Thunder* , despite its best efforts to unbalance us, had been conquered with a mix of humour, courage, and a whole lot of team spirit. As I moved on to the next challenge, I couldn't help but revel in the afterglow of our collective triumph over the circus of chaos that was *Tumble Thunder* .

Having just navigated the wobble-fest of *Tumble Thunder* , the Fab4 now stood before the next epic challenge: *Top of the World* . This was less of an obstacle and more of a height competition on performance-enhancing steroids. Imagine, if you will, two towering wall-like frames set at a 30-degree angle, looming over me like stern, vertically inclined gatekeepers of the heavens. The left frame was designed with a little more consideration for accessibility, while the right frame was reserved for those who fancied a bit of wall-climbing drama, or, as I dubbed it, "the manly wall."

The golden rule for *Top of the World* was as straightforward as it was strict: no lifting or pushing. This was a test of pure climbing prowess, where the only thing being lifted was my spirits—and perhaps the occasional mood after a spectacular stumble. The stakes were high—literally. I am talking about a 12-foot ascent that would make even the most vertically ambitious among us reconsider their choices.

Rohit, with the swagger of a man who had trained for this moment since learning to walk, stepped up to the wall with a confidence that could only be described as majestic. With a powerful leap and a generous application of elbow grease, he scaled the 12-foot frame on his very first try. The crowd—comprised mainly of us—erupted into cheers, and I captured Rohit's victory for posterity with the enthusiasm of a sports commentator narrating a game-winning goal.

With a series of attempts that included everything from impressive ascents to spectacular falls, I finally reached the end of *Top of the World* . My performance may not have been flawless, but my spirits were high, buoyed by my shared camaraderie and the refreshing sips of Red Bull and water that had become our lifeline through the obstacle course. As I continued on, the memory of my escapades at *Top of the World* was a testament to my collective spirit. The obstacle course had tested my limits and given me a series of unforgettable moments.

As the Fab4 strolled their way through the various obstacles with a blend of grace, clumsiness, and pure comedic flair, I arrived at our seventh challenge: *Stack Attack* . This obstacle was like something ripped from the pages of an ancient Greek training manual, minus the togas, amphitheatres, and questionable diet of olives and feta. Stack Attack was, quite literally, a game of "how flexible can I get without making my chiropractor's phone number a staple in my contacts?" Imagine this: a setup with water below, towering vertical frames standing as if they were guarding ancient treasures, and your mission was to manoeuvre with your hands in front and feet behind or shuffle sideways with your back pressed firmly against the wall. It was a gravity-defying dance-off where balance and agility were key.

Promila, ever the daring adventurer, was the first to dive into Stack Attack challenge. With a determined look that said, *"I've got this!"* she launched herself into the task. The result? A splash so grand it could have been mistaken for a scene from a blockbuster water park commercial. Water flew in every direction as if she were auditioning for the role of an aquatic superhero. We cheered and laughed, knowing that Promila's splash would be the stuff of legend—or at least the highlight reel of our event's video footage.

Next up, Aashna and Rohit decided to transform Stack Attack into their personal acrobatic showcase. They turned this seemingly mundane obstacle into a high-flying circus act that had us all questioning whether they had secretly trained with trapeze artists. Aashna leapt onto the top of the frame with such finesse that she seemed to defy gravity. Rohit followed suit with a "casual cool" demeanour that made me wonder if he was strolling through his living room rather than navigating an obstacle course. And then it was me - I approached Stack Attack with the nonchalance of someone casually heading out for a Sunday picnic. My approach was so laid-back that it felt like I was simply strolling through the park, admiring the scenery, rather than tackling a high-stakes obstacle.

With the hilarity of Stack Attack behind me, the next obstacle on my obstacle-riddled agenda was something called *Rise & Grind*. This one was the perfect cocktail of climbing, rope skills, and a touch of grace under pressure—all while trying to avoid an unceremonious splash into the water below. It was like a high-stakes game of 'don't get wet' with a dash of acrobatics thrown in for good measure. It was like being in a reality show where agility, strength, and a bit of flair for the dramatic were your best allies.

Standing tall at 6'2", I tackled the *Rise & Grind* like it was second nature, as if I was built for this climb. Reaching the landing zone? Piece of cake. A quick hop, skip, and jump, and I was there, leaving the rest of the crew watching in admiration at how effortlessly I made it look. But the rope descent? Now, that's where things got interesting. What should've been a smooth slide down the rope turned into something more... artistic. My supposed 'graceful' descent quickly morphed into a sort of rope choreography—a mix of ballet moves and a silent mantra of "please don't fall now!" The crew watched with equal parts amusement and awe as my descent became more of an acrobatic spectacle. When I finally hit the ground, I had earned myself a new badge of honour: a bruise on my left calf, which I rubbed with pride, grinning at my latest battle scar.

In the midst of my obstacle extravaganza, I was suddenly joined by a familiar face: Anirban, a seasoned obstacle runner and fitness enthusiast who had earned his stripes on courses far more challenging than this. His arrival was like a breath of fresh air—if that breath came with the promise of someone else taking on the harder challenges for me. However, true to his enigmatic style, Anirban pulled off a disappearing act worthy of Houdini himself. One moment, he was there, ready to tackle the next challenge with me, and the next—*pff*—he was gone! I was left scratching my head and wondering if I'd somehow master the art of pulling a supersonic speed mid-course. Wherever he went, I wished him Godspeed, and a safe return to the finish.

With the first 8 obstacles behind me, my spirits were as high as ever. Sure, I had my fair share of bruises, wet socks, and hilariously awkward moments, but I'd also shared endless laughter and camaraderie with my group. I knew I had seven more challenges ahead, each promising to push me further, test my balance, and, of course, provide even more opportunities for epic tumbles and side-splitting laughter.

As I marched toward the next set of obstacles, I couldn't help but exchange grins. Whatever came next, I was ready—or at least as ready as I'd ever be. After all, with the Fab4 on the case, what could possibly go wrong?

With the adrenaline from my earlier triumphs still pumping through my veins, I charged ahead to our ninth challenge: the infamous *Rope 'n' Roll*. This obstacle was like a carnival ride designed by someone who had watched way too many action movies. It involved scaling a steep set of steps before launching myself down a slick slide that led straight into a pool of water below. The experience was the perfect mix of exhilaration and refreshment—a bit like diving into a giant, water-filled Popsicle, if that Popsicle was also trying to see how many screams and giggles it could elicit from me on the way down.

The game plan was simple: climb up the steps, throw caution to the wind as I slid down, and then make the biggest splash possible. The water at the bottom was like a cool oasis after a desert trek, beckoning me to dive in with abandon. Each slide turned me into human water missiles, and with every splash, I added to the chorus of laughter and squeals that echoed around the obstacle course. The *Rope 'n' Roll* wasn't just a challenge—it was my opportunity to let loose, channel my inner kid, and fully embrace the joyful chaos that comes with careening into a pool of water with my friends.

Next up was the *Balance Blitz*, an obstacle that should have come with a warning label: "Proceed at your own risk—dignity not guaranteed." It was a horizontal platform suspended by chains over a body of water, wobbling like a new-born giraffe trying to find its legs. This challenge was less about strength or speed and more about not looking like a flailing windmill while trying to keep my balance. The platform had a mind of its own, swaying and tilting with every step I took. It felt as though it was secretly amused by my attempts to cross it without falling into the water below. I wobbled like a toddler in oversized shoes, each step a gamble between staying upright and taking an unexpected dip. It was a circus act waiting to happen, with each of us taking turns attempting the *Balance Blitz*with varying levels of success.

As we regrouped, dripping but undeterred, the next challenge loomed before us: *Swing & Fling*. This obstacle was the ultimate test of my inner primates, a jungle gym for grown-ups where Tarzan himself would have felt right at home. The mission was to climb a rope, swing onto a series of monkey bars, and then somehow make it to the other side without losing my grip—or my dignity.

Aashna, ever the adventurer, was first to take on the *Swing & Fling*. With a burst of energy, she grabbed the rope and swung with a determination that was almost elegant—emphasis on almost. Halfway through her monkey-bar manoeuvre, things took a turn for the dramatic. Her grip faltered, and in a moment of glorious slow-motion, she slipped and fell into the water below, executing a splash so grand it was as if she was auditioning for a part in an epic aquatic movie. The splash was accompanied by a perfectly timed scream that echoed across the course, earning her a round of applause and a few sympathetic winces. Her reward? A bruised knee and shoulder—battle scars she wore with pride as she joined me on the sidelines, laughing off her watery misadventure.

Rohit and Promila, tackled the *Swing & Fling* next. Watching them was like witnessing a pair of trapeze artists at the peak of their game. They swung, leapt, and glided across the monkey bars with the kind of ease that made the rest of us both admire and resent them at the same time. Rohit seemed to have prepared himself perfectly engineered for this kind of challenge, while Promila's agility was on full display. They made the whole thing look effortless, leaving the two of us to cheer them on while secretly hoping they might slip just once to prove they were human after all.

The next up the ante were *Muddy Madness Trio*: *Beat the Drum, Spin Shot,* and *Mud Mayhem*. These obstacles were like an exclusive invitation to the messiest, most chaotic spa day imaginable—minus the cucumber slices and soothing background music, but with a whole lot more sloshing, slipping, and face-planting.

First up was the *Beat the Drum,* an obstacle that sounded innocent enough until I got up close. A giant, mud-filled drum that I had to roll through, emerging on the other side like I'd been caught in a mud storm. It was less of a "roll" and more of a "flop," as I tumbled and slid my way through the drum, completely at the mercy of gravity and the gloopy mess inside. When I finally crawled out, I looked like abstract art pieces—modern, muddy, and with a touch of "I've been through the wringer." My previously distinguishable features were now buried under layers of mud, making me look like living, breathing sculptures ready for a contemporary art exhibition.

Next came *Spin Shot,* a devious concoction of rotating muddy obstacles designed to test not just my agility, but my ability to laugh at myself. The moment I stepped into the obstacle, it was clear that staying clean wasn't an option. *Spin Shot*was like a funhouse ride that had gone rogue, determined to transform me into a human canvas. I tackled it with a mix of determination and reckless abandon, knowing full well that every misstep would result in yet another splash of mud on my already unrecognisable self. But by this point, what was a little more mud? I was practically one with the Earth.

And then, just when I thought I'd reached peak muddiness, I was faced by *Mud Mayhem,* the grand finale of this trio. If the previous obstacles were about getting muddy, this one was about *becoming* mud. The entire course was a mud bath, a playground where the only rule was to embrace the mess. I slid down slopes, slipped over obstacles, and wallowed through the thick, squelching mud like pigs in paradise. Each step felt like a battle against quicksand, with the mud determined to keep me in its sticky embrace. By the time I crawled out, I was no longer an individual but four lumps of living, breathing mud, barely distinguishable from the rest of the Fab4 members.

My muddy adventure was more than just an obstacle course—it was an exercise in letting go. I let go of my need to stay clean, my attempts to look cool, and any hope of avoiding a face full of mud. Instead, I embraced the chaos, revelling in the sheer absurdity of it all. My clothes were beyond saving, my face was smeared beyond recognition, but my spirits? Higher than ever. The sight of the four of us, struggling to climb out of the mud pit, covered head to toe in muck, was the kind of scene that could turn a bad day into a great one.

As I stood there, laughing at the sheer ridiculousness of the situation, it hit me: this was why I did it. It wasn't about the obstacles themselves, but about the shared experience, the camaraderie, and the joy of embracing the unexpected together. *The Muddy Madness Trio* wasn't just about getting dirty—it was about getting lost in the moment, about turning something messy into something memorable.

So, with mud in places, I forged ahead, ready for the ultimate final course.

And then, there it was—the grand finale, the coup de grâce, the challenge that made all the others seem like warm-up exercises for toddlers: *Brain Chiller*. Just the name was enough to send shivers down my spine, but the reality was even more chilling—literally. A towering, slippery incline leading up to a slide that would drop us straight into a pit filled with 4.5 feet of ice cubes. That's right—20 tons of ice, ready and waiting to turn us into human popsicles.

As I stood at the top of that ominous slide, the air was thick with anticipation and, let me be honest, a healthy dose of dread. I paused for a moment, frozen in time, my expressions a mix of excitement and sheer terror. Someone joked about capturing this moment for my future memoirs—if I survived, that is. The thought of plunging into an icy abyss wasn't just exhilarating; it was downright terrifying. I was about to experience a level of cold that could make a polar bear think twice. And then, there was no turning back. One by one, we took the plunge. As soon as I hit the slide, gravity did the rest, and before I knew it, I was hurtling toward the pit of doom. The moment I hit the ice, it felt like being dunked into a frozen blender. Tiny, jagged ice cubes attacked my skin from every angle, while the icy water shocked my system into a state of hyper-alertness. It was as if Mother Nature had decided to drop me straight into the Arctic Circle, minus the snowsuits.

Emerging from the ice pit was like being reborn—except colder and with a newfound appreciation for warm blankets and hot cocoa. I was a chaotic tangle of shivering, gasping, and fluttering limbs, my body in full rebellion against the icy onslaught. Laughter bubbled up uncontrollably, only to be interrupted by chattering teeth and the occasional gasp for breath.

But just as I was about to celebrate surviving the *Brain Chiller*, my attention snapped to Aashna. She was clutching her face, and to my horror, blood was trickling from her lips. For a split second, the laughter stopped, replaced by a surge of concern. Was this the end of our icy adventure? Had the *Brain Chiller* claimed its first casualty? Rushing to her side, I quickly realised that Aashna's injury, while dramatic, wasn't as serious as it first appeared. A minor mishap during the plunge had caused a small cut, but nothing that couldn't be handled with some TLC and a warm towel. The relief was palpable, and we collectively let out a sigh, followed by nervous chuckles. It was a stark reminder that even in the midst of all the fun, safety was no joke. But leave it to Aashna to turn a moment of panic into another badge of honour—after all, not everyone can say they've bled for their sport while conquering an ice-filled abyss.

As I wrapped up my icy ordeal, the adrenaline was still pumping, and despite the freezing temperatures, I couldn't stop grinning. I had conquered *Brain Chiller*, the final, bone-chilling obstacle of the day, and lived to tell the tale. The experience left me with memories (and bruises) that would last a lifetime, along with a newfound appreciation for the warmth of the Sun and the simple joy of dry clothes.

So, with the final challenge behind me, we huddled together, shivering and laughing, ready to toast to our victory—not with champagne, but with the promise of hot showers and even hotter stories to share. Because if there was one thing the Fab4 knew how to do, it was to turn even the iciest of challenges into a reason to celebrate.

But hold on—my adventure was far from over! As the Fab4 regrouped, I noticed that Promila was MIA. In true Fab4 spirit, Aashna, who had recently returned to the fray, took it upon herself to locate her partner in crime. This wasn't just a search mission; it was like embarking on a scavenger hunt through a maze of obstacles and cheering crowds.

After a quick round of *"Where's Promila and now Aashna?"* and *"Has anyone seen them?"* I decided to launch my own search mission. And what did I find? Promila and Aashna, who had apparently decided that an obstacle course was the perfect backdrop for a Bollywood dance-off. Yes, you read that right. The girls had traded their muddy shoes for dancing feet and were shaking it to some seriously infectious Bollywood beats. Their energy levels were so high they could have powered a small city. Promila was executing some elaborate dance moves that could only be described as "impressively enthusiastic," while Aashna had fully embraced the role of the Bollywood diva. I caught them mid-twirl, and after a quick chat and a hearty laugh, I informed them about their new mission: rendezvousing with Rohit at the baggage counter.

Speaking of Rohit, it turned out he had been busy too. After securing the bags, I attempted to catch up with him, only to find him in the midst of a mini workout frenzy. Apparently, he had ventured into the competitive zone and was on the brink of conquering 700 squats. Yes, you heard that right—700. Talk about beast mode! Despite his heroic efforts, Rohit's lower body seemed to be on strike after the epic squat session. But did that stop him from posing for the paparazzi? Absolutely not! With a smile and a flex, he showed off his accomplishments, proving that he could still deliver the goods in front of a camera even if his muscles were ready to file for retirement.

Meanwhile, Aashna and Promila, undeterred by their earlier Bollywood escapades, decided to dive into a burpee battle with a couple of other girls. The competition was fierce, the stakes were high, and the sweat was pouring. Drumroll, please! Aashna, with the determination of a warrior and the endurance of a marathon runner, emerged victorious. She cranked out 70 burpees and was rewarded with a shiny pair of cool earphones. It was like winning the fitness lottery, and Aashna wore her prize with the pride of a true champion.

I, slightly bemused by the frenetic energy of Aashna, Promila, and Rohit, decided it was time for a breather. I found a cozy spot to catch my breath and reflect on the day's events. It was a moment of calm amidst the chaos—a chance to appreciate the sheer absurdity of the adventures and the boundless enthusiasm that had fuelled us. With hunger pangs now clawing at our stomachs, we made our way to Adayar Ananda Bhavan for a hearty lunch. We devoured our meals with the enthusiasm of people who had just completed a marathon. The food was a well-deserved reward, and we ate like there was no tomorrow. Reflecting back, I embraced the challenges, laughed at the mishaps, and made every step of my journey a celebration of friendship and fitness. So, here's to more adventures, more obstacles, and more moments of pure, unadulterated fun with the best crew you could ask for.

Tee-Rific Triumph: The 5:30 AM Squad's Epic Tee-Shirt Adventure

On Feb 19, 2024, as usual, the gym was a hive of sleepy chatter and shuffling footsteps. Friends exchanged bleary-eyed greetings, their voices muffled by the thick, woolly layers they'd wrapped themselves in against the cold. In the midst of this morning ritual, Neelima and Niharika, two of the earliest risers, were huddled together, trying to shake off the last vestiges of sleep.

"Wouldn't it be amazing," Neelima said, her voice a mix of stifled yawns and excitement. *"If we had t-shirts that screamed 'I'm a part of this epic Early-Morning Club'?"*

Niharika, rubbing her eyes and trying to focus on the vision Neelima had just painted, responded with a sleepy grin, *"Yeah, and imagine the look on people's faces, when we roll-in wearing them. We'd look like the coolest, most committed team in the gym!"*

Their conversation, like most pre-workout chats, began with half-hearted enthusiasm but quickly gained momentum. As Neelima and Niharika tossed around ideas about their potential gym attire, I, who had been warming up in my own corner, caught wind of the conversation.

I, ever the early riser (used to now!) and always on the lookout for the next big idea, couldn't resist chiming in. My eyes lit up with the kind of enthusiasm that suggested I had just stumbled upon a revolutionary concept.

"T-shirts?" I exclaimed, my voice brimming with excitement. I clapped my hands together with the exuberance of a kid who'd just found out his birthday party was going to be at an amusement park. *"That's genius! Let's make this happen!"*

The simple notion of custom t-shirts quickly began to snowball, fuelled by the morning's caffeine and the endorphins from their workout. What started as a casual musing over the cold, hard gym floor, evolved into something much more substantial. My energy was like a spark igniting a powder keg of creativity and enthusiasm. Before long, we three were buzzing with ideas. We debated colours, designs, and slogans with the fervour of true visionaries.

"We could go for something bold," I suggested, my mind racing with possibilities. *"Something that says, 'We're not just early risers; we're a team that's up before the world!'*

Neelima, already envisioning the potential impact, added, *"Yes, we could have our own unique slogan – something that captures our dedication and spirit."*

Niharika, caught up in the whirlwind of excitement, was practically vibrating with anticipation. *"Let's do it! Let's make these t-shirts happen!"*

The conversation, initially just a bit of pre-workout banter, had transformed into a full-blown project. Our knack for turning dreams into reality meant that this wasn't going to be just a passing whim. The idea was gaining momentum, and soon, the entire crew was buzzing with excitement about their new venture. The t-shirt project wasn't just about the fabric and ink—it was about creating a symbol of our commitment, camaraderie, and early-morning resolve. My enthusiasm was contagious, and it wasn't long, before the casual idea had turned into a mission. With every enthusiastic shout and brainstorming session, the project took shape, promising to become an epic chapter in our early-morning saga.

As the spark of the t-shirt idea spread through the 5:30 a.m. workout crew, it was clear that this wasn't a task I could tackle solo. To turn this vision into reality, I needed a dream team—a squad of enthusiastic and skilled individuals who could handle everything from brainstorming to execution. The project was quickly evolving from a simple idea into a full-fledged mission, and I knew I needed the right people on board to make it a success.

First on my list was Mahesh (our '*Krishna*'), my reliable right-hand man. If there was a gold medal for multitasking, Mahesh would have it hanging proudly around his neck. Known for his legendary organisational skills, Mahesh was the guy who could keep a dozen spinning plates in the air without breaking a sweat. His uncanny ability to manage resources and juggle tasks made him the perfect candidate to handle the logistical side of the project. Mahesh's reputation as a problem-solver preceded him. When I approached him with the t-shirt idea, his eyes lit up with the kind of excitement usually reserved for discovering a new workout routine. "*I'm in,*" Mahesh said, barely pausing between sips of his morning coffee. "*Let's make these t-shirts happen!*"

Next up was Ravina, the detail-oriented maestro of coordination. If Mahesh was the project's logistical engine, Ravina was the finely-tuned GPS system that kept everything on track. Known for her impeccable organisational skills and ability to manage ideas with a level of precision that bordered on the obsessive, Ravina was like the glue that held the team's creative visions together. I knew that with Ravina on board, the project would benefit from her knack for keeping everyone aligned and focused. "*I'm ready to dive in,*" Ravina said, her enthusiasm tempered by a look of meticulous determination. "*I'll make sure we hit every milestone without missing a beat.*"

Realising that the project needed a touch of artistic flair, Arjun extended an invitation to Promila, a professional designer with an eye for the extraordinary. Promila was the kind of designer whose portfolio was filled with jaw-dropping creations that made you question how you ever lived without her work in your life.

When Promila joined the team, she brought with her a whirlwind of creativity and innovation. Her first question was, *"What's the vibe we're going for?"* With her expertise in design, Promila was tasked with translating the team's vision into something that would not only look amazing but also embody the spirit of the 5:30 a.m. crew.

To round out the team, I brought in Sudhakar and Anand. Sudhakar was known for his out-of-the-box thinking, often proposing ideas that left others scratching their heads in both wonder and confusion. His knack for innovation meant that the t-shirt project would benefit from his unique perspectives and inventive solutions. Anand, on the other hand, was the creative powerhouse with an ability to think beyond conventional boundaries. His ideas were as unconventional as they were brilliant, and his enthusiasm for the project was infectious. Together with Sudhakar, Anand promised to add a layer of creativity that would set the t-shirts apart from anything the gym had ever seen.

The first official meeting was held at a cozy local café, a favourite spot for many post-workout hangouts. The café, with its inviting aroma of freshly brewed coffee and the sight of healthy snacks laid out on the counter, was the perfect setting for brainstorming. As the team settled into their seats with steaming cups of coffee, the energy in the room was palpable.

I kicked off the meeting by laying out the vision for the t-shirts.

"We need something that's more than just a piece of clothing," I said, leaning forward with a look of determination. *"We need t-shirts that scream '5:30 AM Crew' and which embodies the spirit of our group."*

Mahesh nodded, already envisioning the logistical challenges ahead.

"We'll need to decide on the material, find a reliable vendor, and figure out how to get these shirts produced in bulk." Added Ravina, ever the detail-oriented planner. *"I'll keep track of all the ideas and make sure we stay on schedule. We don't want to miss any deadlines."*

Promila, with her designer's eye already working overtime, asked, *"What kind of design are we looking at? Classic, modern, or something completely out there?"*

Sudhakar and Anand exchanged glances, their minds already whirring with creative possibilities. Sudhakar said, *"How about incorporating elements that symbolise our commitment and unity? Maybe a design that tells a story?"*

Anand chimed in, *"We could also use some unique slogans that capture our early-morning spirit. Something that resonates with everyone and adds a personal touch."*

As the discussion flowed, it became clear that the project was taking shape. Ideas were tossed around, debated, and refined. The café buzzed with excitement as the team began to lay the groundwork for what would become their signature t-shirt.

To keep everyone in the loop and streamline communication, I created a dedicated WhatsApp group, aptly named '*Fit Buddies – The Apparel Crew*'.

The group quickly became the central hub of activity, with messages buzzing back and forth like a hive of creative bees. In this virtual space, the team shared ideas, sketches, and updates. The group chat was a flurry of activity, with everyone contributing their thoughts and feedback. I wanted to make sure that the group's collective energy is committed to making the t-shirt project a resounding success. The WhatsApp group became a place where ideas were brainstormed, decisions were made, and the team's camaraderie was strengthened. It was here that the initial excitement of the project was transformed into actionable plans, and where the vision of the t-shirts began to take concrete shape.

The first challenge with the team's quest was to create the perfect t-shirt was selecting a colour. Now, one might think that choosing a colour is a straightforward task. Ha! Think again. The colour debate was nothing short of an epic showdown, a spectacle of decision-making that could rival any high-stakes poker game. As the team gathered for their first brainstorming session, the mood was a mix of excitement and sleep-deprivation-induced giddiness. Coffee cups were stacked high, and the air was buzzing with the kind of energy that only comes from the combination of caffeine and creative chaos. The team was ready to tackle their first big decision: colour.

"Okay, folks," I began, *"What's our colour?"*

"Red!" Mahesh chimed in, almost too eagerly.

"No way," Promila shot back, waving her hands as if swatting away an imaginary mosquito. *"Red is so… loud. We need something more understated."*

"Black," Ravina suggested, raising an eyebrow. *"It's classic, versatile, and slimming. Plus, we all want to look like we're auditioning for a superhero movie, right?"*

A chorus of *"Yes!"* and *"Absolutely!"* rang out, and just when it seemed like black was going to be the unanimous winner, Anand piped up.

"But black can be so… predictable. What about teal?" Anand proposed, his voice filled with the kind of optimism that only comes with the belief that teal is the next big thing.

A moment of silence fell over the group. It was as if everyone was collectively pondering the existence of teal and whether it truly belonged in their colour palette.

"Teal?" I echoed, scratching my head. *"We're not exactly launching a Caribbean cruise line here."*

As the debate raged on, it became clear that choosing a colour was not just about aesthetics but about creating a statement. The team discussed visibility, personal preferences, and the potential of each colour to flatter various body types. By the end of what felt like a marathon discussion, it was decided.

"Black it is!" I declared with a dramatic flair. *"Classic, versatile, and slimming. We're basically going to look like a squad of superheroes."*

The team cheered, relieved that the colour decision was finally behind them. Little did we know, the real fun was just beginning. With the colour settled, the team dove headfirst into the design process. If we thought choosing a colour was intense, designing the t-shirts was akin to participating in a high-stakes game show, where creativity and humour were the ultimate prizes.

Over the next three weeks, the team met regularly. We gathered in our usual café, turning napkins into makeshift canvases and brainstorming sessions into lively debates. Every meeting felt like an episode of a reality TV show, complete with plot twists, dramatic reveals, and spontaneous dance breaks.

"We need a design that screams 'We're Awesome!'" Promila said, waving her hands as if conducting an invisible orchestra.

"Agreed!" Sudhakar nodded enthusiastically. *"But we also want something that reflects our unique spirit. Something that says- 'We're cool, but we're also approachable.'"*

"Like a unicorn riding a rainbow?" Anand suggested, clearly not missing a beat.

"Unicorns are so last year," Ravina countered. *"We need something fresh and original. How about a design that incorporates our team's commitment and unity?"*

The room erupted into a flurry of sketching, doodling, and laughter. Napkins were covered in scribbles, and coffee stains became unintentional art pieces. Ideas were tossed around like confetti, with each member adding their own flair to the mix.

At one point, someone proposed incorporating our Fitness Centre logo into the design. The room fell silent, and eyes turned towards me.

"Hold on," I said, raising a hand. *"We don't want to end up in court over a t-shirt!"*

"Good point," Mahesh agreed, nodding sagely. *"We should avoid any potential legal drama."*

So, with a collective sigh of relief, we decided to put the wordings: *'Fit Buddies'* and below it, the slogan- *"Challenge Your Limits."*

With the decision made to go original, our vision for the t-shirt design began to take shape. I had a grand idea involving a constellation of stars and a rising horse. The idea was as unique as it was ambitious.

Picture this: a constellation featuring a rising horse, with stars ascending from the bottom right to the mid-chest area of the shirt. The stars symbolised our unity and individual strengths, while the horse represented our journey and growth. It was a design that was meant to be both striking and meaningful.

I shared my vision with the team, and Promila, the artistic genius among them, took the reins. With a flair for artistic expression and a knack for translating ideas into stunning visuals, Promila got to work.

"Alright, let's get this design rolling!" I announced, with excitement evident in my voice.

Promila began sketching, her pencil moving with a fluidity that made it seem like she was channelling her inner artist. The initial sketches were filled with energy and imagination, capturing the essence of my vision. As Promila worked on refining the design, the team watched in awe. The constellation began to take shape, with stars twinkling and the rising horse becoming a symbol of their collective journey. It was clear that the design was evolving into something truly special.

The team's meetings became a blend of creative brainstorming and laughter. We reviewed the progress, made suggestions, and occasionally indulged in impromptu dance breaks to keep the energy high.

"I think we need more stars," Promila said during one review. *"The design needs to really pop."*

As the design neared completion, the team couldn't contain their excitement. They eagerly discussed the placement, colours, and final touches. The rising horse, now surrounded by a constellation of stars, was turning into a design that was as unique as their group.

The design was nothing short of a masterpiece. The constellation of stars, ascending gracefully to form the rising horse, symbolised their unity and individual strengths. The slogan "*Challenge Your Limits*" was proudly displayed, reminding everyone of their commitment to pushing boundaries and striving for greatness.

As the team admired the creation, it was clear that the design was more than just a t-shirt. It was a representation of our 5.30 a.m. crew journey, our camaraderie, and our shared passion for fitness. It was a design that would become a symbol of our early-morning dedication and our unwavering spirit. With the design finalised, the team prepared for the next steps. The excitement was palpable as we looked forward to seeing our creation come to life. The t-shirts were not just a piece of apparel—they were a testament to our hard work, creativity, and the bond we had formed along the way. And so, with the design ready and the team's enthusiasm at an all-time high, the journey continued. The t-shirts were about to become a reality, and the team couldn't wait to see their vision come to life.

Once the design was ready, it was time to pick the fabric. The team knew we needed a fabric that could withstand our rigorous workouts while keeping us comfortable and stylish. After all, if we're going to sweat buckets, we might as well do it in a fabric that won't make us feel like we're wearing a sauna suit.

"Alright, folks," I declared, channelling my so-called inner fashion guru. *"We need a fabric that's breathable, durable, and comfortable. We want to look good and feel good, no matter how many reps we're pumping out."*

"Dri-fit!" Mahesh suggested, waving a swatch of fabric as if it were a magic wand. *"It's perfect for all our needs."*

"Dri-fit sounds like a winner," Ravina agreed, nodding with enthusiasm. *"It wicks away sweat and keeps us looking fresh. Plus, it sounds way cooler than 'moisture-wicking'."*

With the decision made, our team embarked on the vendor hunt, our first stop being a warehouse that looked like it had been plucked straight out of an old-school adventure movie. Dusty and dimly lit, it had the ambiance of a place where treasure might be hidden—or where old t-shirts went to die.

"Welcome to the T-shirt Dungeon!" the vendor greeted them with a grin. *"What are you looking for?"*

"We're on the hunt for high-quality dri-fit fabric," I replied, trying to look as professional as possible while secretly wondering if I'd accidentally walked into a time warp.

The vendor led us through piles of fabric swatches, each one more colourful and questionable than the last. Mahesh took to examining samples with the precision of a scientist, while Ravina jotted down notes as if she were compiling a secret dossier. After what felt like an eternity of inspecting fabrics and negotiating prices, the team stumbled upon a vendor offering good branded t-shirts. The quality was top-notch, and the brand name added an extra layer of coolness that made everyone's eyes light up.

"A branded t-shirt!" I exclaimed, as if I'd just discovered the Holy Grail of t-shirt fabrics. *"This is perfect!"*

However, the excitement was short-lived when we saw the price tag. At *Rs.1499* per t-shirt, it was a bit steep for our budget. We huddled together, strategizing our next move.

"Okay, we need to negotiate," Anand said, rolling up his sleeves with the determination of a gladiator entering the arena. *"I've got this."*

Anand, with his charm and persistence, took centre stage. The negotiation process resembled an intense poker game, with Anand using every trick in the book to bring down the price. The vendor, impressed by Anand's persistence, started to crack.

"Look, we're ordering a bulk quantity," Anand said, flashing his most convincing smile. *"We need a better price if you want this deal to happen."*

The vendor raised an eyebrow, clearly intrigued by Anand's offer. *"Alright, what's your offer?"*

"Rs.500 per t-shirt," Anand said confidently, as if he were making the most reasonable offer in the world.

The vendor's eyes widened. *"That's quite a drop from Rs.1499. Are you sure?"*

"Absolutely," Anand replied, his charm and confidence radiating like a superpower. *"We're committed to this project, and we need your support."*

After a tense few minutes, the vendor relented. *"Alright, you've got a deal. Rs.600 per t-shirt, provided you order at least 40 units."*

'Yes!' Anand accepted. *"And we would need a sample t-shirt!"*

The team erupted into cheers, celebrating our victory as if we'd just secured a major sponsorship deal. The savings were significant, and the t-shirts were now within our budget.

"Looks like we're in business!" I exclaimed, high-fiving Anand. *"You've done it again."*

The day we were all waiting for, had finally arrived—April 12, the day when months of brainstorming, negotiating, and dreaming would culminate in a grand unveiling. It was the day when the first sample t-shirt would make its debut at the workout session, and Mahesh was the chosen bearer of this monumental garment.

Mahesh strutted into the gym with the kind of confidence usually reserved for superheroes making their entrance. Clad in the sample t-shirt, he looked like he was ready to take on the world—or at least, the next set of burpees. The moment he walked in, all eyes were on him, and a collective gasp of awe escaped the crowd.

"Ladies and gentlemen," Mahesh announced, striking a dramatic pose. *"Behold, the t-shirt that will change our workout lives forever!"*

The design was even better than they had imagined. The fabric, a perfect blend of comfort and style, hugged Mahesh's physique in all the right places. The vibrant '*Fit Buddies*' wording shimmered with a promise of sweat, camaraderie, and the occasional post-workout brunch.

"Wow," Niharika exclaimed, her eyes wide with admiration. *"It's like it was tailor-made for us!"*

As everyone admired the sample, the initial shock of the t-shirt's retail price of Rs.1499 quickly evaporated when I revealed the miraculous discounted price of Rs.600 per t-shirt. Gasps of relief and joy filled the room as if everyone had just won a jackpot.

"Rs.600!?" Neelima exclaimed, practically bouncing off the walls. *"That's a steal! I'm want five of them!"*

With the t-shirt's official debut a resounding success, it was time to get serious about placing orders. I created a Google Form to collect everyone's t-shirt requests. The form was simple: name, size, and quantity. What could go wrong? Well, apparently, nothing. The response was overwhelming. The Google Form practically exploded with orders. Within a day, we had 25 orders, and by the end of the week, we had hit the magical number of 40. It seemed like everyone was eager to get their hands on the new gear. Some members were so enthusiastic that they ordered multiple t-shirts, presumably to make sure they had a fresh one for every day of the week—or just to flaunt their fitness pride. Ravina took charge of tracking the orders and payments with the precision of a well-oiled machine. Her spreadsheets were a marvel of organisation, and she made sure that not a single order was misplaced or forgotten. It was like watching a maestro conduct a symphony of t-shirt transactions.

As the delivery date approached, the excitement was palpable. The WhatsApp group, affectionately named '*Fit Buddies – The Apparel Crew*,' was abuzz with updates and countdowns. Each day brought a new flurry of messages, emojis, and exclamation points.

"Only three more days to go!" someone would post, followed by a flurry of celebratory emojis.

"Can't wait to see the t-shirts!" another would chime in, with a gif of a person dancing in anticipation. The group chat had become a hive of excitement, with everyone eagerly anticipating the arrival of their new gear. It was as if they were waiting for a shipment of gold bars or the latest must-have gadget.

May 17 arrived, and with it, the moment they had all been waiting for. Mahesh, having donned the mantle of the unofficial 'T-shirt Distribution Czar,' picked up the consignment from the vendor. The sight of the neatly packed boxes filled with the new t-shirts was like opening a treasure chest. Mahesh carefully sorted the t-shirts by size, labelling each one with the respective member's name. It was a meticulous process, but one that was executed with a sense of pride and joy. The t-shirts looked even more fantastic in person, and it was clear that all our hard work had paid off. The workout crew gathered for the grand distribution, and the excitement was electric. As each member received their t-shirt, the air was filled with cheers, high-fives, and a few spontaneous dance moves. It was a moment of triumph and camaraderie, a celebration of their collective effort and enthusiasm.

"Check it out!" Neelima said, twirling in her new t-shirt. *"I feel like a superhero!"*

"Look at this design!" Promila exclaimed, showing off the t-shirt to anyone who would listen. *"It's like wearing a badge of honor!"*

As the distribution continued, it was clear that the new t-shirts were more than just workout gear. It was a symbol of our group's unity and our shared journey. The excitement was palpable, and the sense of pride and accomplishment was undeniable.

The morning after the grand distribution was nothing short of epic. The gym was abuzz with energy as the 'Fit Buddies' strolled in, each one proudly sporting their new t-shirts like they'd just received an honorary degree in fitness fashion. The atmosphere was charged with a sense of accomplishment that could rival the excitement of a rock concert.

Mahesh, always one to seize the moment, suggested they commemorate the occasion with a group photo.

"We need to capture this!" he declared, his voice ringing with the gravity of a major historical event. *"It's our moment of glory!"*

The group assembled in their t-shirts, striking poses that ranged from the classic 'Power Stance' to the more daring 'Pretend we're Superheroes' look. The camera clicked away, capturing a series of photos that would later be remembered as some of our finest work. As the flashbulbs went off, Neha couldn't help but remark, *"I'm pretty sure we're about to become Instagram famous. I can already see the hashtags: #FitBuddies #TShirtGoals."*

As the new t-shirts made their debut, the gym quickly became a hotbed of conversation. The 5:30 a.m. crew had effectively turned into the gym's coolest new trendsetters. Other members couldn't resist approaching them with a mix of admiration and curiosity.

"Hey, where did you guys get those shirts?" asked one intrigued early riser, eyeing the t-shirts like they were the latest must-have gadget.

"Oh, these?" I responded with a grin. *"They're a special edition. Designed by us, for us. It's a long story – one involving a lot of caffeine and negotiations."*

The gym-goers were fascinated. The 'Fit Buddies' were no longer just another group of early-morning exercisers. They had become the talk of the gym, embodying a sense of unity and style that turned heads and sparked conversations. The success of the t-shirts quickly transcended the gym's walls. Friends and family, who had heard whispers of the epic t-shirt saga, were eager to hear the full story. It was as if the t-shirts had become a symbol of something greater—an emblem of creativity, teamwork, and relentless enthusiasm.

My family, in particular, was intrigued. They peppered me with questions about the design, the process, and the negotiations. *"It sounds like you've been through an adventure!"* my daughter exclaimed. *"Can I get one of these t-shirts too?"*

And so, the t-shirt story became a cherished tale, retold with pride and enthusiasm at family gatherings, brunches, and even casual meet-ups. The journey from brainstorming to the grand reveal had captured everyone's imagination, and the t-shirts had become a symbol of our collective effort and triumph. The impact of the t-shirt project went beyond mere aesthetics.

"Look at us!" Promila exclaimed during a particularly intense session. *"We're like a well-oiled fitness machine, only with more style!"*

The t-shirt project had not only brought us closer as a group, but also added a whole new layer of fun to our routine. Every time we wore those t-shirts, it was a celebration of our shared achievements, and a reminder of the laughter and challenges we had faced together. The Fit Buddies sported their tees with pride—not just because they symbolised fitness, but because they represented a journey packed with creativity, negotiation, and just the right amount of madness. These shirts weren't just about accomplishments; they embodied our collective spirit.

'Fit Buddies' became a sense of identity. We were no longer just a bunch of people showing up at the gym at the crack of dawn; we were a unified team with a shared mission and a distinctive look. The t-shirts had turned our early-morning grind into a memorable adventure. During workouts, the crew now moved as a coordinated unit, our matching t-shirts serving as a reminder of their shared journey. It was as if the fabric itself was infused with the spirit of their camaraderie and hard work.

Embracing Responsibility with a Dash of Fun

It was April 21, 2024, Koramangala, Bengaluru. The air buzzed with a blend of excitement and pre-workout jitters. I was eager to dive into the day's events. Roshni, our resident fitness aficionado, had set the stage for what promised to be an epic fitness odyssey. She had created a WhatsApp group named 'Fit Champs', and today, that group was about to leap from the digital realm into the physical world.

As I and others gathered at the Fitness Centre, the atmosphere felt charged, like the opening scene of a blockbuster movie. Today, a select few would be celebrated as 'Fit Champs' for the hard work we'd all invested in our fitness journeys. When the clock struck 11:20 a.m., I stepped into the workout arena, my heart racing with anticipation for the surprises that lay ahead. Entering this fitness battleground, I scanned the room for familiar faces amid the crowd of eager, pumped-up fitness enthusiasts. It was like arriving at a big party and searching for someone you know, hoping to find a touch of familiarity to ease your nerves and break the ice.

So, who were the 'Fit Champs'? According to our Fitness Centre, they're not full-blown trainers but rather friendly guides on this thrilling fitness voyage. They're there to cheer us on, offer a helping hand, share a smile, and provide a pep talk when our muscles are begging for mercy.

Roshni, the mastermind behind this campaign, was our leader for the day. Her mission was to unite the chosen Fit Champs and imbue them with the wisdom of Cliff Robertson's iconic Spiderman line: "*With great power comes great responsibility.*"

Prahar, my fitness guru with a charisma as magnetic as his workouts, kicked off the session with warm-ups that could double as a mini workout in it's own right. The group of to-be adorned Fit Champs stretched, jumped, and wobbled their way into the groove, the bodies slowly warming up to the challenges ahead. As if sensing the group's growing excitement (and perhaps our impending exhaustion), Prahar introduced our first workout: *Rock Paper Scissors.* Sounds like a game your toddler might play, right? But oh no, this was the grown-up, adrenaline-pumping version.

Roshni divided the group into two teams of 20, armed with nothing but barbell plates and a burning desire to win. The objective? Arrange those plates into an 'S-shape' and hop on them from start to finish. Simple enough, except the hopping part made me feel like a caffeinated kangaroo in a tutu. The team that managed to hop, would outwit the opponent in *Rock Paper Scissors,* and reach the last dumbbell plate first, would be the champions of this whimsical workout.

It sounded straightforward when explained, but the reality was more akin to a circus act with a dash of gym madness. A chaotic scene with people hopping, slipping, and occasionally toppling over like bowling pins. After a lot of hopping and a few bruised egos, a victorious team emerged (sadly, it wasn't mine). We congratulated them, our faces redder than a beetroot from the exertion and laughter.

With my initial energy spent and my spirits high, I dove headfirst into the next challenge: the *Circuit Workout*. This was not for the faint-hearted. Again, the group was split into teams of five and faced a series of tasks that would make even the most seasoned fitness fanatic break a sweat:

- ***Pull-ups:*** At least one member had to complete 10 reps, while others hung from the bar like very sweaty decorations.
- ***Goblet Squats:*** 30 reps of squatting while holding a weight like you're about to win the World's Strongest Man competition.
- ***V Sit-ups:*** 30 reps of trying to look like a well-practiced ballet dancer while lying on the floor.
- ***Deadlifts:*** 30 reps of lifting and lowering weight with the grace of a robotic penguin.
- ***Side-to-Side Shuffle:*** 30 reps of shuffling side-to-side as if you're dodging invisible obstacles.
- ***Plank Drags:*** 30 reps of dragging a weight while holding a plank, trying not to collapse into a heap.
- ***Push Presses:*** 30 reps of pressing weight overhead, all while pretending you're lifting a small planet.
- ***Burpees:*** 30 reps of the most comprehensive workout move known to mankind, combining a squat, a jump, and a push-up into one sweaty extravaganza.

As I faced the *Circuit Workout,* I couldn't help but think I hadn't signed up to be the next Arnold Schwarzenegger or Sylvester Stallone. But with my regular workouts at our Fitness Centre, I'd built some solid strength and stamina. It wasn't about transforming into a superhero overnight; it was about embracing the challenge and giving it my all. Each member cheered each other on, bonded over a collective struggle, and celebrated every tiny victory. After what felt like an eternity of grunting, sweating, and laughing, I finally reached the end of the day's adventures. The cooldown session was a welcomed oasis of tranquility, a soothing balm to my exhausted muscles. As I stretched and breathed deeply, my fatigue was tempered by the satisfaction of having given it my all.

The grand finale of our 'Fit Champs' extravaganza came with a tangible symbol of our efforts: the coveted 'Fit Champ' t-shirt. Roshni and Prahar stood proudly, showcasing how taking on responsibilities could be both challenging and incredibly rewarding. The t-shirt was more than just a piece of apparel; it was a badge of pride, a symbol of my dedication and camaraderie. As I donned my new 'Fit Champ' gear, I couldn't help but feel a sense of accomplishment. The day had been a whirlwind of laughter, challenge, and triumph. I had embraced the journey, supported each other through every hurdle, and emerged stronger—both physically and mentally.

So, here's to Roshni for orchestrating this fitness fiesta, to Prahar for keeping me motivated, and to all the 'Fit Champs' who made this day unforgettable. Our adventure wasn't just about fitness; it was about building connections, pushing boundaries, and discovering that with a little bit of grit and a lot of laughter, anything is possible.

Epilogue: The Fitness Journey Continues…

As I close the final pages of this book, I'm reminded that fitness is so much more than a series of exercises; it's a dynamic, multifaceted adventure filled with motivation, strength, flexibility, and community. Each chapter—from those early Tuesday morning bursts of inspiration to our grand escapades—has woven together a narrative that truly captures the essence of lifelong fitness.

I've come to realise that fitness isn't just about shaping my body; it's about evolving both as an individual and as part of a community. Those early days as a Fit Buddy were rich with lessons—not just from my own progress, but from the shared experiences of those around me. I discovered the power of encouragement, the joy in collective triumphs, and the importance of viewing every hurdle as an opportunity for growth.

My transition from Fit Buddy to Fit Champ wasn't a single moment of victory, but a continual commitment to the journey. As I took on more responsibility—not only for myself but also in supporting others—I realised that true strength lies in helping others rise, just as much as in lifting weights.

The best is yet to come, and with every step, I'm becoming stronger, more resilient, and more connected. I embrace this lifelong adventure of fitness and camaraderie, allowing it to enrich my life in ways I had never imagined.

As I continue on my own fitness journey, I hope the stories and insights in this book serve as a guide for you. May they ignite your motivation, give you the courage to face new challenges, and inspire you to build a supportive network around you.

Here's to the many adventures still to come, the sweat and laughter yet to be shared, and the incredible community of fitness enthusiasts who make every moment of this journey truly rewarding. The adventure is far from over, and the most exciting chapters are still ahead.